KETO CLEANSE

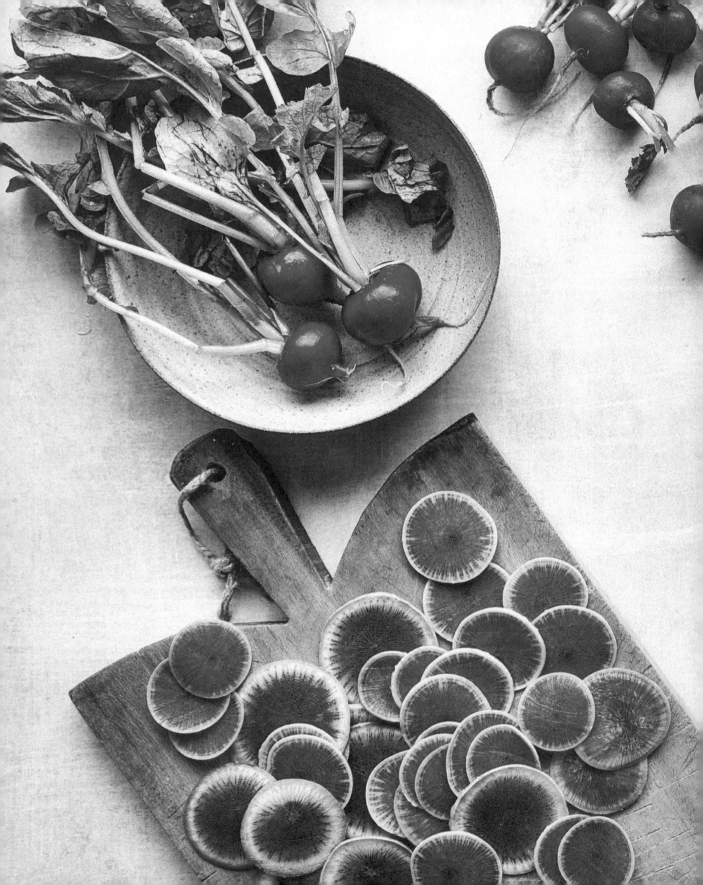

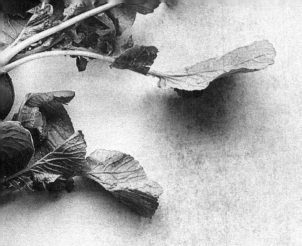

KETO CLEANSE

14-Day Plans to Reset with a Clean Ketogenic Diet

KARISSA LONG

ROCKRIDGE
PRESS

Interior and Cover Designer: Matt Girard

Photo Art Director/Art Manager: Sue Bischofberger

Editor: Rachel Feldman

Photography © 2020 Hélène Dujardin. Food styling by Anna Hampton.

Author photo courtesy of Alexandra Strimbu.

ISBN: Print 978-1-64611-648-5 | eBook 978-1-64611-649-2

R0

To anyone looking for a clean start, may this book inspire you to take the first step. I promise you, you won't regret it!

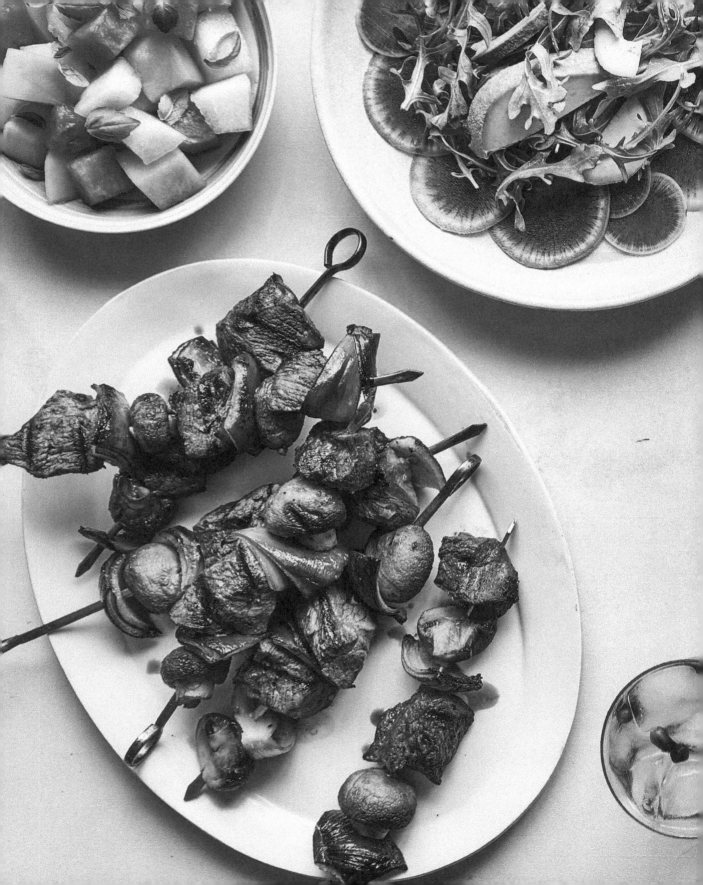

CONTENTS

INTRODUCTION

I have to admit, I have a love–hate relationship with the term "cleanse."

Most people associate cleanses with deprivation, restriction, and starvation. And for the most part, they're right. Many mainstream cleanses require you to drink juice, tea, or some other liquid at every meal for several days in an attempt to remove toxins from your body.

Well, I'm here to tell you that these types of cleanses are a bad idea—they're not enjoyable, feel like punishment, and can actually be unhealthy for your body. Those juices and teas may provide some vitamins and minerals, but they also deprive you of vital macronutrients your body needs in order to function properly. It's also worth noting that drinking liquids all day doesn't actually remove toxins from your body. Yep. That's actually the responsibility of your organs and immune system.

So, what *should* you do if you're trying to "cleanse" your body? It's simple: Focus on *supporting* the health of your organs and immune system, which are responsible for detoxing the body. The best way you can do that is to feed your body the nourishing, nutrient-dense whole foods that are essential for optimal wellness. When you give your body what it needs to function well, it will not only "cleanse" itself—it will also thrive!

On that note, I welcome you to the *Keto Cleanse.* This book centers on cleanses that follow ketogenic diet principles and are designed for nourishment, satiation, and enjoyment. That's right—you will nourish your body from the inside out with a menu of healthy fats, quality protein, and organic vegetables. This is a cleanse that you'll actually enjoy.

As a global health coach and ketogenic expert, I have been living the keto lifestyle for almost a decade. I found the ketogenic diet during my battle with ulcerative colitis. Within a few months on the diet, I shed my excess weight, gained more energy, improved my focus, started sleeping better, improved my skin, and managed my cravings, and—to my surprise—my autoimmune disease went into remission.

The improvement in my quality of life created a passion to help others do the same. I launched a company, Clean Keto Lifestyle, devoted to helping people transition into a sustainable keto lifestyle so that they, too, can thrive. I love the work I do and I'm proud to say that since starting my company, I've helped thousands of people achieve their health goals with a ketogenic way of life.

Although I have been living this way for years, I'm not perfect. At times, I find myself eating too many keto-friendly treats, eating out nightly, and indulging in one too many adult beverages (tequila on the rocks with lime is my go-to). When that happens, I feel sluggish, moody, and simply not my best self. That is when I know I need a reset—we all do every once in a while.

So, I wrote this book to provide you with an easy plan to do just that. In the following chapters, I explain my philosophy on ketogenic cleanses, detail the steps you should take to get prepared, provide you with three 14-day meal plans designed to be enjoyable *and* easy to implement, and share over 100 delicious and nutritious keto recipes perfect for anyone looking to give their body a fresh start. By the end of this book, you will feel confident, prepared, and, most importantly, *motivated*.

To a clean start,
Karissa

PART ONE

Clean Keto Reset

A clean keto reset is unlike any type of cleanse you have tried before. We're doing things differently this time. First and foremost, we're following the principles of the ketogenic diet. This way of eating completely changed my life and transformed my health for the better, and I know it can do the same for you. Second, we are focusing on all the foods that *you can eat* versus focusing on what you can't. This simple mind-set shift makes a huge difference. And finally, we are going to be eating delicious meals that will not only nourish your body, but also satiate it—meaning absolutely no starvation and no punishment! Are you ready to start healing your body from the inside out?

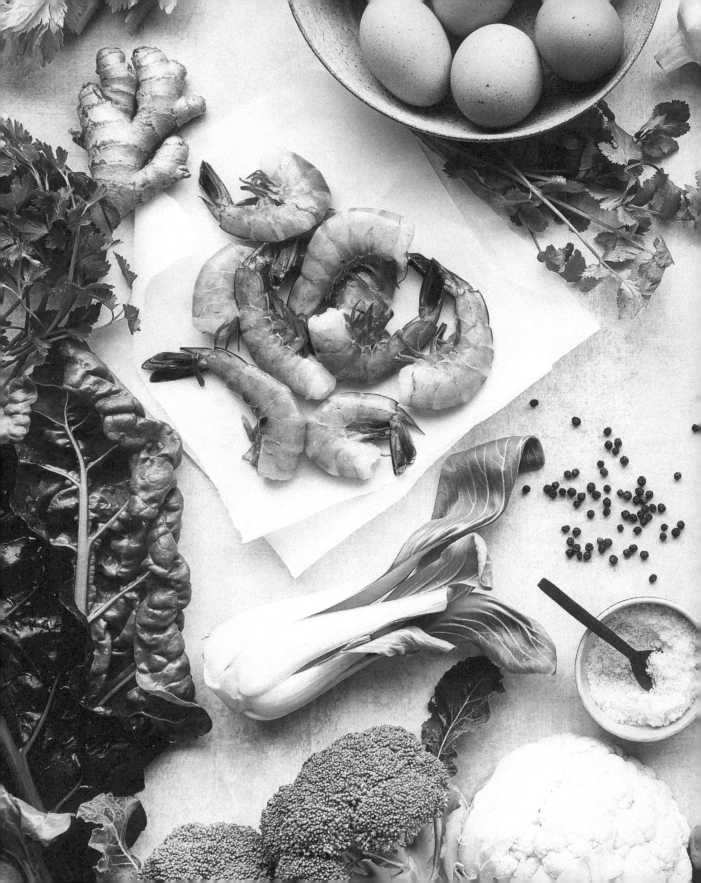

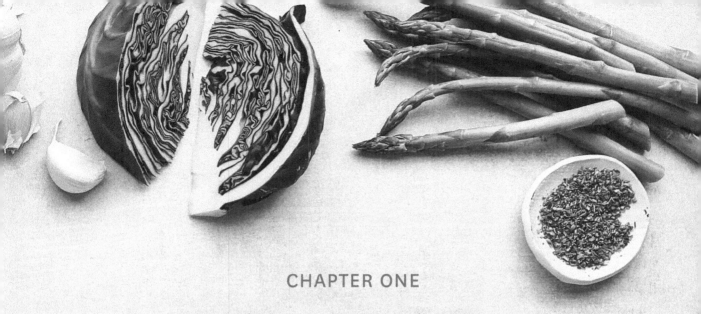

CHAPTER ONE

Healing with Keto

I have been helping people master the ketogenic diet and reset their bodies for a long time now, and what I have found is that knowledge *truly* is power. If you are informed, you are empowered to make good decisions. If you know how certain foods affect your body, then you can choose wisely and feel confident in your choices.

This chapter provides all the information that you need to be successful. I break down all the basics, including why cleanses are beneficial for your body, why keto makes a great diet to cleanse with, and why my cleanses are so effective and enjoyable.

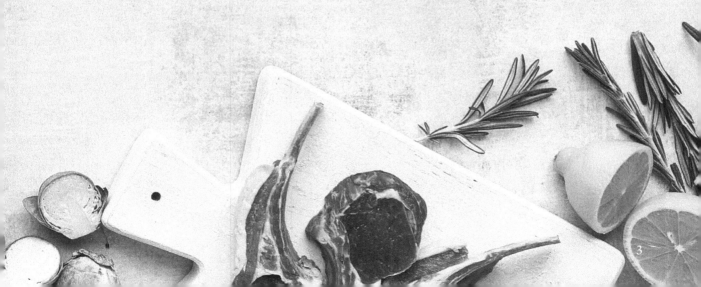

Going on a Cleanse

A cleanse essentially means a process or period of time where you're actively trying to rid your body of toxic or unhealthy substances—which are abundant. Every day, your body is exposed to chemicals, bacteria, pathogens, viruses, and other toxins. They lurk in your food in the form of pesticides, herbicides, antibiotics, and GMOs. They lurk in your homes in the form of cleaning products, skincare items, paint, furniture, and carpeting. They exist in your water supply in the form of chlorine, lead, and even arsenic. Fortunately, your body is equipped with a sophisticated detoxification system to handle these toxins. This system includes the following:

Immune system: An intricate system made up of multiple organs and thousands of cells that work collectively to fight off invaders and remove them from your body.

Liver: Home base for detoxing. The liver allows nutrients from food to enter your bloodstream while quarantining toxins and excreting them into your bile, which eventually flows into the intestines to be eliminated.

Colon: Lined with cells that help block harmful substances from moving into your bloodstream. Regular bowel movements eliminate these substances before they can harm you.

Lungs: Your body's air purifiers. They filter out damaging particulates and vapors. Tiny filaments called cilia line your airways and help prevent pollutants from passing into your bloodstream.

Kidneys: Filter all the blood in your body and dispose of toxins in your urine every 35 to 45 minutes.

The key to properly detoxing your body is to ensure that these organs and systems are working efficiently. Unlike most cleanses, which can deprive you and force your body into starvation mode, the goal of my keto cleanses is to provide your body with an abundance of nutrient-dense, whole foods designed to nourish these detoxifying systems so they can do their jobs more effectively.

When your body is functioning optimally, its ability to detoxify improves. As a result, you begin to look and feel amazing! The first time I did one of the cleanses in this book, I noticed a significant improvement in my energy levels, experienced less bloating, had glowing skin, and slept like a baby. Bottom line: I felt rejuvenated from the inside out.

Because my cleanses are all about nourishment, you could eat like this every day for the rest of your life if you wanted to. But I want you to live your life and not feel the pressure to be perfect all the time. I recommend using the cleanses in this book in whatever way works best for you, whether that means as an occasional reset or on a regular basis. The choice is yours. At the end of the day, as I always say, everyone is different. You know your health and dietary needs better than anyone else. When in doubt, always consult your doctor before trying something new that you're unsure of.

Cleansing with Keto

What exactly *is* keto, and how can it help cleanse the body? The ketogenic diet is a low-carb, moderate-protein, high-fat diet designed to exhaust glucose levels and prompt the body to provide an alternative source of energy to the brain. These alternative energy sources are called ketones. These ketones are produced in the liver from stored fat in the body. When your body is in a state of ketosis, it literally becomes a fat-burning machine, and burning fat is a great way to cleanse your body for a few important reasons:

1. Fat cells house pollutants and chemicals, so every time you burn stored fat cells for fuel, you also remove those stored toxins. By being in ketosis, you can naturally detox your body.

2. Fat burning, and the resulting weight loss that occurs, also has positive effects on your liver and metabolic health, which is critical for your body's detoxification. Your liver is involved in virtually every metabolic process in the body, including ridding your body of toxic substances. Excess weight puts undue stress on your liver, and when your liver is overburdened, its ability to function is hindered. As you release excess weight, your liver and its detoxication functions improve.

THE THREE CLEANSES IN THIS BOOK

I know what you're thinking—and no, you won't be eating lettuce for 14 miserable days! I've made it my mission to ensure that the meals you will eat taste incredible and keep you satisfied. You probably won't even think twice about what's missing from your plate because you'll fall in love with all the amazing ingredients you're enjoying instead.

I know from working with my clients that everyone has varying needs, which is why I designed three distinct cleanses for this book.

1. THE KETO CLEANSE

This cleanse is rooted in clean, ketogenic principles to get you into and/or maintaining ketosis. Each meal contains only whole foods: nothing processed, no artificial ingredients, no chemical additives. On this cleanse, you'll avoid the following food categories, which have been associated with digestive issues, intolerances, and sensitivities.

GRAINS: Including wheat, barley, rye, spelt, oats, and buckwheat. These foods are high in carbohydrates so they can spike your blood sugar and hinder your body's ability to get into ketosis. Also, the lectins found in grains are hard to digest and have been shown to lead to intestinal permeability.

GLUTEN: Gluten is a family of proteins found in most grains. Gluten allergies, sensitivities, and intolerances are becoming more common because gluten is difficult for your body to digest. It can also damage the gut lining, which compromises your body's ability to absorb nutrients.

DAIRY: Including milk, cheese, butter, cream, yogurt, and whey. The main carbohydrate in dairy is lactose, a milk sugar that many people can't properly digest. In fact, a majority of the world's population suffers from lactose intolerance. People who are lactose intolerant can suffer from chronic digestive problems if they continue to consume it. *I do have one dairy exception in this book: ghee.* Technically, ghee is not dairy-free as it is derived from butter, but it is lactose-free because all the milk solids are removed, making it much easier to digest. It's also high in healthy fats and fat-soluble vitamins like A and E so a few of the cleanse recipes will include this ingredient.

SWEETENERS: Although sugar-free sweeteners like stevia, monk fruit, and erythritol are keto-friendly, they can cause digestive distress for some people. They're also mainly used in keto desserts and treats that don't provide much nutritional value.

2. THE ELIMINATION CLEANSE

This cleanse takes the Keto Cleanse a step further. Two food categories that are often problematic for people (especially those suffering with autoimmune or digestive conditions) will be eliminated: nuts and seeds and nightshades. After eliminating these food categories for 14 days, you can assess how you are feeling and if you should reintroduce them.

NUTS AND SEEDS: For some people, nuts and seeds cause gastrointestinal distress because they contain a large quantity of phytic acid, which binds to minerals like zinc, iron, magnesium, calcium, chromium, and manganese in the gastrointestinal tract. These bound compounds generally cannot be absorbed in the intestine and as a result can impair digestion. One exception to seeds are seed-based spices, such as mustard seed and cumin seed. Most people can tolerate small servings of seed-based spices, so they are used in limited quantities during the Elimination Cleanse.

NIGHTSHADES: Including eggplant, peppers of all kinds (bell peppers, hot peppers, paprika, cayenne), tomatillos, and tomatoes. Although the majority of people have no issues with nightshades, they can cause problems for some people, especially those with autoimmune conditions or chronic digestive issues. This could be attributed to the fact that nightshades are high in lectins and alkaloids, both of which can aggravate the gut. Spices from the nightshade family contain capsaicin (one of the chemicals that give them heat), which is a potential gut irritant for some people, so these are eliminated in this cleanse as well.

3. THE INTERMITTENT FAST CLEANSE

This cleanse mimics the Keto Cleanse but changes your eating schedule. This meal plan will utilize the 16:8 method of intermittent fasting, which requires restricting your daily eating period to 8 hours and fasting for 16 hours in between. During the fasting period, you can still consume water, unsweetened tea, black coffee, and bone broth. See page 17 for more on intermittent fasting.

3. The transition from burning carbs as fuel to burning ketones can initiate and increase autophagy in your body. Autophagy means "self-eating," and is your body's natural way of removing damaged cellular components and replacing them with new ones. It is the ultimate detox for your body and can improve your body's natural ability to function.

Getting into ketosis comes down to the specific macronutrients (or macros) you eat and in what proportion. There are three types of macronutrients: fat, protein, and carbohydrates. On the ketogenic diet, your daily macronutrient breakdown should be as follows:

75% fat   **20% protein**   **5% carbohydrates**

That's right—about 75% of what you eat each day comes from fat. Fat is the most essential macronutrient the body needs. You need fat to live, and it is necessary for you to get into ketosis.

The amount of each macro you're consuming is important, but what you're consuming to make up those macros is equally important—and that's where "clean" keto comes into play.

BENEFITS OF THE KETO CLEANSE

Before you embark on a keto cleanse let's review the numerous benefits:

WEIGHT LOSS AND FAT BURNING. By definition, being in a state of ketosis means you are burning stored fat for energy. Weight loss happens quickly and can be significant, because you are turning your body into a fat-burning machine when you are producing ketones.

INCREASED ENERGY LEVELS. This occurs as a result of your body running on a more efficient fuel source in the form of ketones. Ketones are able to cross the brain's blood barrier to provide consistent and superior energy, which (compared to glucose) means your energy levels will skyrocket.

IMPROVED BRAIN FUNCTION. Other than fat loss, another big reason so many people turn to the ketogenic diet is for improved mental clarity; to finally lift that brain fog once and for all. In fact, a sharper mind is normally one of the first benefits you notice when achieving ketosis. This is because (compared to glucose), ketones are an upgraded fuel source for your brain. Studies have shown that ketones can provide as much as 70% of your brain's energy needs and are more energy-efficient than glucose.

CONTROLLED APPETITE. One of the most profound benefits of the ketogenic diet is the fact that you aren't hungry all the time and you don't experience cravings for sugar. When you burn ketones as fuel rather than glucose, your blood sugar levels are stabilized.

RELIEF FROM/REVERSAL OF SYMPTOMS OF SOME AUTOIMMUNE CONDITIONS. Your digestive system and gut microbiome play a huge part in your immune system and in autoimmune disease. The ketogenic diet promotes the healing of your gut lining because you are ridding your body of inflammatory grains and sugars. This healing combined with the keto diet reducing inflammation overall can make it an effective tool for reversing the symptoms of autoimmune conditions.

INCREASED VITAMIN AND MINERAL CONSUMPTION. Fat plays a crucial role in vitamin and mineral absorption. It needs to be present when ingesting fat-soluble vitamins (A, D, E, and K) so that they are properly absorbed by your body. Because you consume 75% fat when eating keto, your body's ability to absorb vitamins and other nutrients significantly increases. When you couple this improved absorption with all the nutrient-dense vegetables and proteins you consume on a clean keto diet, you'll find that you have an effective formula for restoring your body's essential vitamins and nutrients.

OTHER BENEFITS. My clients have also reported better sleep, less acne, improved skin conditions, better muscle tone, and a balanced mood after adopting a ketogenic diet, which makes them look and feel younger. Research also links the ketogenic diet to a multitude of other benefits, including cancer treatment and prevention, reduction in chronic disease, Alzheimer's treatment, neuroprotection, and brain trauma injury healing.

My Clean Keto Philosophy

Unfortunately, with the growing popularity of keto also comes misinformation, clever marketing by food companies, and improper implementation. I mean—*it is not all about bacon and cheese!*

I believe the key to implementing the keto diet the right way is to focus on one important principle: food quality. By feeding your body the highest-quality foods, you provide the nutrients it needs for its detoxification system (and all of its systems, for that matter) to function optimally.

A clean keto diet is rooted in the principles of whole foods. That means you remove low-carb processed foods, refined oils, chemical additives, and factory-farmed meat and seafood from your plate, and instead, load it up with the nutrient-dense real foods that nourish your body.

What makes this approach to keto so effective is that it is based on the way your body was built to perform at its best. When you eat healthy fats, quality protein, and organic vegetables, your body recognizes them and can digest them easily. By filling your plate with food of the highest standard, you will restore and revitalize your body.

HEALTHY FATS

There are many different varieties of fat, ranging from healthy to downright dangerous for you (i.e., trans-fat and hydrogenated oils). Because the ketogenic diet focuses around fats, it is vital that you consume the right ones. The fats you ingest should come from whole, unrefined foods such as olives, avocados, and coconuts. Healthy fats should come from the farm—not factories—and have no added ingredients. When available, opt for organic versions to limit your exposure to GMOs, pesticides, herbicides, and other toxins.

QUALITY PROTEIN

Eating quality protein is critical for everyone, regardless of what diet you consume. Conventional protein sources today (meat, poultry, eggs, and seafood) that are the most widely available to consumers are also most likely mass-produced, factory-farmed, and unhealthy for you. Most of these animals (even the fish!) are raised in conditions that are overcrowded and dirty. To control disease, these animals are pumped full of antibiotics and other pesticides. They are also fed a grain-based diet, which results in inflammation, depleted nutrients, and high instances of omega-6 fatty acids (the bad kind, if too high) in the animals. Remember, at the end of the day: "You are what your food eats."

That's why it's absolutely necessary for your health to eat the most nutrient-dense, quality protein available. My definition of quality protein means sourcing and consuming grass-fed beef, pastured poultry and eggs, heritage-breed pork, and wild-caught seafood. It is 100% worth the extra effort and money to find and purchase quality protein. (See Sourcing High-Quality Ingredients on page 23.)

ORGANIC VEGGIES

Organic vegetables make up the majority of all the carbs you consume on the ketogenic diet. You need to eat vegetables on keto to ensure that you are getting sufficient fiber, vitamins, and minerals. When picking your vegetables, opt for the non-starchy variety and make sure they are organic whenever possible. Organic produce is grown and processed without bioengineered genes (GMOs), synthetic pesticides, petroleum-based fertilizers, and sewage sludge-based fertilizers. Organic vegetables have higher antioxidant, vitamin, and mineral content than their conventionally grown counterparts. Often, when people with intolerances to chemicals or preservatives switch to eating only organic vegetables, they find that their symptoms lessen and even go away.

Foods to Eat and Avoid on Keto

The following charts will act as your reference guide throughout the cleanses. There are four sections:

Foods to eat freely: These are meant to be eaten in abundance. Opt for the highest-quality and the most nutrient-dense foods available (see page 23 for what you should look for on the labels).

Foods to eat in moderation: These are foods that have a higher carbohydrate and sugar content. Your daily intake should be limited to ensure that it doesn't hinder your ability to achieve and maintain ketosis. The Elimination Cleanse also removes all nightshades, nuts, and seeds included in this category.

Foods to avoid: These foods should be avoided because of their high carbohydrate content or because they promote inflammation.

Foods to avoid initially but can be reintroduced: These foods are removed from your diet as part of the cleanses. All the cleanses remove dairy, sweeteners, and low-sugar alcohol. These categories can be added back in moderation after your cleanse if you can tolerate them.

FOODS TO EAT FREELY

HEALTHY FATS

Avocado	Coconut milk, full-fat	Lard
Avocado oil	Coconut oil	MCT oil
Coconut butter, manna, or cream	Extra-virgin olive oil	Olives
	Ghee	

QUALITY PROTEIN

Beef	Eggs	Scallops
Beef gelatin powder	Halibut	Sea Bass
Chicken	Lamb	Shrimp
Collagen peptides	Pork	Tuna
Crab	Salmon	Turkey

NON-STARCHY VEGETABLES

Arugula	Bok choy	Brussels sprouts
Asparagus	Broccoli	Cabbage

Cauliflower	Kale	Shallots
Celery	Leeks	Spinach
Chard	Lettuce	Sprouts
Chives	Mushrooms	Zucchini
Cucumber	Onions	
Garlic	Radishes	

FERMENTED FOODS

Kefir (non-dairy)	Kimchi	Sauerkraut

HERBS AND SPICES

Basil	Curry	Peppermint
Bay leaf	Garlic	Rosemary
Black or white pepper	Ginger	Sage
Cardamom	Horseradish	Tarragon
Cilantro	Mustard	Thyme
Cinnamon	Nutmeg	Turmeric
Clove	Oregano	Vanilla (powder or
Cumin	Parsley	gluten-free extract)

FLAVORINGS

Capers	Pink Himalayan salt	Vinegars (apple cider,
Coconut aminos		balsamic, red wine, and
Fish sauce		white wine)

BEVERAGES

Bone broth	Unsweetened herbal tea (black,
Seltzer/sparkling water,	green, chamomile, peppermint)
unflavored	Filtered water

FOODS TO EAT IN MODERATION

LOWER-SUGAR FRUITS (MAX ½ CUP PER DAY)

Blackberries	Grapes	Raspberries
Blueberries	Lemon	Strawberries
Cranberries	Lime	Watermelon
Cantaloupe	Peaches	
Grapefruit	Pomegranate seeds	

NIGHTSHADES

Eggplant	Peppers of all kinds (bell peppers, hot peppers, paprika, cayenne)	Tomatillos
		Tomatoes

NUTS (INCLUDING BUTTERS AND MILKS)

Almonds	Macadamia nuts	Pistachios
Brazil nuts	Pecans	Walnuts
Cashews	Pine nuts	

SEEDS (INCLUDING BUTTERS AND MILKS)

Cacao/cocoa	Poppy
Chia	Pumpkin
Coffee	Sesame
Flax	Sunflower
Hemp	

FOODS TO AVOID

GRAINS AND STARCHES

Barley	Oats	Rye
Buckwheat	Quinoa	Wheat
Corn	Rice	

HIGHER-SUGAR FRUITS (INCLUDING FRUIT JUICE)

Apples	Figs	Pears
Bananas	Kiwi	Plums
Cherries	Mango	Pineapple
Dates	Oranges	

STARCHY VEGETABLES

Butternut squash	Potatoes
Plantains	Sweet potatoes

BEANS AND LEGUMES

Beans	Peanuts
Lentils	Peas

HIGH-SUGAR ALCOHOL

Beer	Hard ciders
Dark liquors	Sweet wine

REFINED OILS

Canola	Grapeseed	Soybean
Corn	Margarine	Vegetable

REFINED SUGAR OF ALL KINDS

Agave	High-fructose	White sugar
Brown sugar	corn syrup	
Evaporated cane juice	Powdered sugar	

ARTIFICIAL SWEETENERS AND DRINKS

Energy drinks	Soda/diet soda	Sweet'N Low
Equal	Splenda	Truvia

FOODS TO AVOID INITIALLY BUT CAN BE REINTRODUCED

DAIRY

Butter	Full-fat yogurt	Whey
Buttermilk	Heavy cream	
Cheese	Sour cream	

KETO SWEETENERS

Erythritol (non-GMO)	Monk fruit extract (100% pure)	Stevia (100% pure)

NATURAL SWEETENERS (MAX 1 TEASPOON A DAY)

Coconut sugar (5 carbs per teaspoon)

Molasses (5 carbs per teaspoon)

Pure maple syrup (4 carbs per teaspoon)

Raw honey (6 carbs per teaspoon)

LOW-SUGAR ALCOHOL

Clear liquors

Dry wines

Keto and Intermittent Fasting

Another powerful way to get into ketosis and detox your body is through intermittent fasting. Intermittent fasting is essentially a type of eating schedule that is focused on giving your body an extended period of time between feedings.

After you eat, your body spends the next few hours digesting that food, processing it, and burning what it can as fuel. Your body will take the most readily available energy source for fuel, which is the food you just ate, rather than the fat you have stored. This is especially true if you just consumed glucose (sugars and carbs), as your body prefers to burn glucose as energy before any other source. If you are in a fasted state (you haven't recently consumed a meal), your body doesn't have that readily available glucose as energy, so it is more likely to pull from the fat stored in your body and generate ketones. And, as we know, good things happen when you are in ketosis.

This book includes a cleanse plan that incorporates the 16:8 method of fasting, which requires restricting your daily eating period to 8 hours, while fasting for 16 hours in between.

Here are some of the great benefits to intermittent fasting:

- **Weight loss.** Because intermittent fasting can activate ketosis, it can help you lose weight and belly fat.

- **Simplified meal planning.** Most intermittent fasters skip breakfast, meaning that is one less meal to have to plan, prepare, and eat, which saves both time and money.

- **Healing.** Taking long breaks between meals gives your digestive system a break where it isn't actively trying to process and break down food. This allows your body to rest and heal.

- **Autophagy.** Fasting can also initiate autophagy, which is a cellular regeneration process in your body. Having an extended fasting window gives your body a chance to cleanse itself and eliminate toxin buildup by regularly removing damaged cells and tissues and replacing them with new ones.

WHO SHOULDN'T FAST?

For the most part, the only negative side effect of intermittent fasting is hunger. Most people experience this side effect only in the first few days, while their body is still adjusting to a new way of eating. But intermittent fasting is not advised for the following people:

- Anyone struggling with (or prone to) an eating disorder
- Anyone who has issues with blood sugar regulation
- Anyone who suffers from hypoglycemia or diabetes
- Anyone who is malnourished
- Children under 18 years old
- Pregnant women
- Breastfeeding women
- Anyone taking daily medications that require consumption with food

What to Expect

One of the biggest challenges when starting a cleanse is just that—starting! Many people find themselves stressing out over meal planning, grocery shopping, cooking and prep work, and how to find keto recipes that they'll actually want to eat.

That's why I've done all the work for you by curating three separate keto cleanse plans. Each plan is 14 days long and full of nourishing and delicious foods, shopping lists, and meal prep instructions intended to minimize your time in the kitchen.

With each of the cleanses in this book, we are going to be loading up your body with vitamins, nutrients, and minerals that are intended to restore your health and make you look and feel vibrant. Rather than surviving off of liquids all day (as you do in many typical cleanses) that make you feel hungry, sluggish, and weak, you will enjoy whole foods that both satisfy and satiate you and, most importantly, are designed to get you into ketosis.

In fact, you can expect to get into ketosis within two to seven days of starting the cleanse depending on your current glycogen supply, body type, and activity level. This means you can begin reaping the amazing benefits of ketosis in as little as one week. As you move into the second week of each cleanse, your energy levels should be higher, your mood should be better, and you should be feeling lighter and leaner. By the end of each cleanse, you will feel reset and renewed!

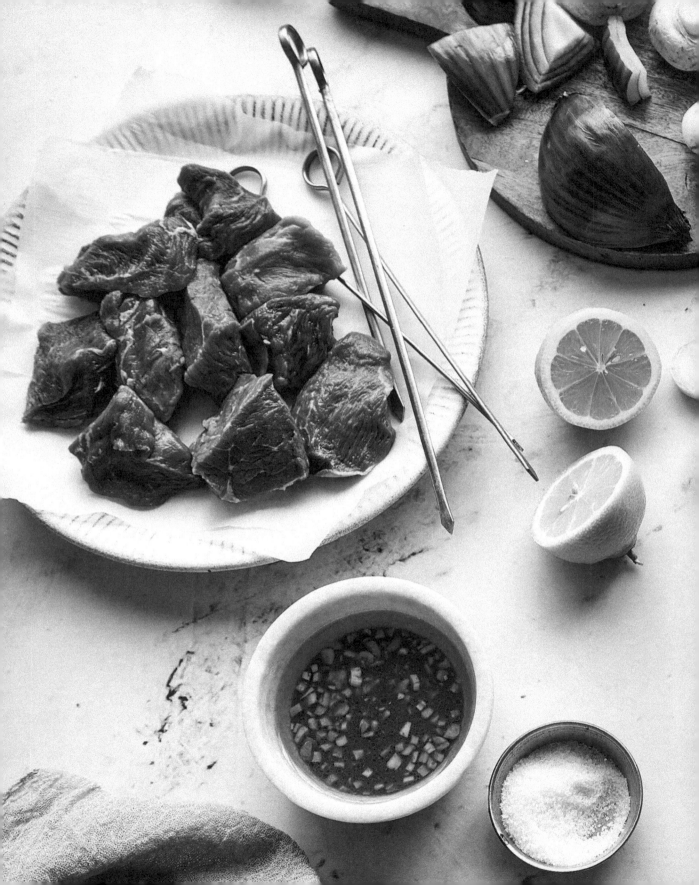

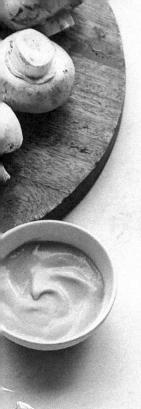

CHAPTER TWO

Preparing for the Cleanse

Before you jump into the keto cleanse plans, you'll need to get organized. I sincerely believe that preparation equals success. The purpose of this chapter is to get you ready for a clean start. I'll show you how to stock your kitchen with essential keto tools and ingredients, what lifestyle changes to make, and the tips and tricks that will make your cleanse as successful as possible.

Stocking Your Keto Kitchen

Having a well-stocked kitchen and the right equipment is essentially all you need to master keto cooking. Let's go over what you need on hand before starting your cleanse.

TOOLS AND EQUIPMENT

Keto cooking doesn't require fancy equipment, but you do need a few basics. You most likely own a majority of these items already.

MUST-HAVES

- Baking sheet
- Blender
- Cutting board
- Food processor
- Grater
- Large stockpot with lid
- Mesh strainer
- Mixing bowls
- Parchment paper
- Saucepan
- Sharp knife
- Skillets (1 small; 1 large)
- Slow cooker
- Steamer basket
- Storage containers (airtight, various sizes)
- Utensils (peeler, spatula, strainer)

NICE-TO-HAVES

- Cast iron skillet
- Spiralizer
- Steamer
- Vitamix (or other high-speed blender)

Sourcing High-Quality Ingredients

To eat quality, nutrient-dense foods, you first need to source them. Make sure to look for the following quality indicators on food labels:

- **Fats:** organic, unrefined, non-GMO

- **Proteins:** organic, grass-fed, grass-finished, heritage-breed, pastured, pasture-raised, wild-caught

- **Vegetables:** organic, non-GMO, local

With that in mind, here are some places to start looking.

Grocery stores. Most grocery stores offer some variety of quality foods. Look in the produce section for certified-organic labels or stickers on the item. All vegetables and fruits have a PLU code. Organic PLU codes have a five-digit number that starts with the number 9.

Cost-Saving Tips:

- **Buy private label.** Most supermarkets offer their own private-label organic food lines. Because there is no middleman, the prices are cheaper. Just make sure you see the certified-organic seal on the item.

- **Take advantage of sales.** Shop the circulars and look for the yellow sale tags, which often indicate a product is on sale.

- **Buy in bulk.** When it comes to nuts, seeds, and even meat, buy them in bulk at a cheaper cost per pound. Portion out what you will use within a week and then freeze the rest in sealed containers. Yes, even the nuts and seeds should go in the freezer and will last for up to a year.

Your local farmers' market. You can't beat the taste and nutrient profile of food that comes straight from a nearby farm. The shorter transport time ensures that you are getting the food at its peak freshness. Make sure to seek out farmers who use organic farming techniques.

Cost-Saving Tips:

- **Comparison shop.** Walk the entire market before you make any purchases and compare the prices and quality between the vendors.

- **Buy seasonal produce.** Fruits and vegetables that are in season are generally the most affordable.

- **Shop near closing.** Some vendors will discount their prices right before closing time in order to off-load their produce rather than reload it back onto their trucks.

Shop online. Shopping online is a great option if you can't find quality foods at your local grocery store or farmers' market. It's also a good option for busy people who don't have the time to go to the store each week and enjoy the convenience of getting food shipped directly to their front doors.

Cost-Saving Tips:

- **Shop discount websites.** There are many websites that offer quality products at affordable prices. My favorites are:
  - Amazon
  - Thrive Market
  - Butcher Box
  - Sizzlefish
  - Now Foods

- **Sign up for offers.** When prompted, provide your email address so you can sign up to get notified when there are sales or promo codes.

Success on the Cleanse

The following tips are what I use in my life to stay on track, and also what have worked well for my clients. They are realistic, straightforward, and easy to implement, and I urge you to put these into practice as well.

GET MENTALLY PREPARED

Before starting any of the cleanses, there are a few things you need to do in terms of mind-set. Checking these items off your list will properly prepare you and your mind for the upcoming journey.

Figure out your "why." Before starting anything in life, you should understand why you are doing it. So ask yourself, why do you want to embark on a cleanse? Write down all your "whys" and put them in a place where you will see them daily.

Pick a date. Timing makes a big difference when you're about to embark on a cleanse. There are usually two types of people: Those who like to dive in headfirst into a new way of eating and those who need to ease into it slowly.

If you're diving in:

- **Clear your calendar.** Look for a 14-day window that makes sense for you to start. You are looking for a low-stress time frame that allows you time to cook meals at home and focus on yourself. That means you want to avoid starting the diet when you have a huge deadline at work, are busy with kids' activities, or are going on vacation. No time is ever perfect, but try to identify a realistic start time.

If you're easing into it:

- **Week 1:** Aim to remove processed food from your diet. Don't worry about macros—just make sure you are eating real food.

- **Week 2:** Aim to eliminate sugars from your diet—cane sugar, honey, maple syrup, agave, and other natural sweeteners. This will slowly start to lower your carb count.

MOVE CONSISTENTLY

Regular physical movement is a fantastic way to support metabolic function, improve digestion, lift your mood, and boost your energy. The great news is that you don't need to spend hours a day in the gym to see results. Here's my movement strategy:

- **Consistent low-impact cardio:** Focus on consistent movement every day throughout the day and make it a priority to fit in as much as possible. Go for a refreshing walk in the mornings and evenings, park in the farthest spot from the entrance, or go to a yoga or Pilates class.
- **Shorter high-intensity workouts:** Add 30 minutes of high-intensity workouts three or four days a week. Do sprint intervals, high-intensity interval training workouts, dance cardio, swimming, or cycling.

MANAGE STRESS

Chronic and consistent stress can lead to health problems such as internal inflammation, hormone imbalance, and a weakened immune system. Here are some great ways to relieve stress: practice meditation, get a massage, take a relaxing bath, pick up a relaxing hobby (painting, knitting, or gardening).

SLEEP WELL

Sufficient sleep is a must when you are doing a cleanse. Your body not only needs sleep to function, but it also needs sleep time to repair, restore, and recover. Aim to get seven to nine hours of sleep each night.

- Create a bedtime ritual and follow it each night with the goal of going to sleep at the same time every day.
- Put down your phone and turn off the TV at least two hours before your bedtime to avoid blue light exposure, which can be disruptive to your sleep cycle.
- Improve your sleep environment by making sure your bedroom is quiet, dark, and cool.

ELIMINATE TOXINS IN YOUR ENVIRONMENT

Toxins are also prevalent in household products, personal care items, and water supply. As you breathe these toxins, apply them to your skin, and/or ingest them, you are bombarding your body with chemicals and irritants. Try to eliminate as many toxins as possible from your daily life.

- **SWAP OUT YOUR CLEANING SUPPLIES.** Opt for natural-based cleaning products that use essential oils, vinegar, and other plant-derived ingredients. Here are some brands I trust: The Honest Company (www.honest.com), Seventh Generation (www.seventhgeneration.com), Branch Basics (www.branchbasics.com), and Mrs. Meyers (www.mrsmeyers.com).
- **UPGRADE YOUR SKIN AND MAKEUP PRODUCTS.** Sadly, most skincare, haircare, and makeup companies use harmful ingredients in their products. Here are my favorite places to shop for clean beauty brands: Credo Beauty (www.credobeauty.com), The Detox Market (www.thedetoxmarket.com), Whole Foods (www.wholefoodsmarket.com), and The Honest Company (www.honest.com).
- **FILTER YOUR WATER.** Unfortunately, most standard tap water can be contaminated with toxins such as lead, arsenic, and radium. You can use water filters to protect yourself from potentially harmful contaminants; the most affordable options are water filter pitchers or faucet-attachment filters.

PRACTICE SELF-COMPASSION

Your thoughts tremendously affect how you live your life and being hard on yourself can hinder your ability to succeed. Work to focus on positivity and self-compassion.

- **Quit the negative self-talk.** Bashing yourself takes a toll. When you hear yourself saying or thinking negative thoughts, immediately stop yourself and replace it with a positive comment.
- **Replace limiting beliefs.** Limiting beliefs normally start with the phrases "I can't" or "I will never." Replace these beliefs with aspirational thoughts starting with the phrases "I can" and "I will."
- **Stop resisting change.** If you want different results, do things differently. Make small changes consistently, and they'll add up and transform your life.
- **Pat yourself on the back.** Celebrate your successes. Nothing is too small to celebrate—be proud of yourself every step of the way.

- **Week 3:** Aim to eliminate grains from your diet—bread, pasta, rice, and cereal. Replace these foods with servings of healthy fats and organic veggies. For example, if you normally eat salmon with brown rice, upgrade your meal to salmon pan-seared in avocado oil, served with grilled asparagus topped with extra-virgin olive oil and lemon.

- **Week 4:** You are ready to start the Keto Cleanse!

Stop being scared of fat. In my practice, I often see people who find it difficult to change their mentality toward fat after years of thinking it was the enemy and the cause of weight gain and other health issues. But trust me—healthy fats are the key to managing your appetite, keeping cravings at bay, and getting into ketosis. And good fats won't make you fat! I promise.

Get your mind right. Don't view keto as a short-term fix. Instead, approach keto as a lifestyle change and something you plan to adopt long-term. Focus on your health first and the ability to nourish, heal, and restore your body instead of solely focusing on weight loss. This health-first mind-set makes it much easier to stay motivated.

MEAL PREP

Meal prep is a critical step to success. By planning and prepping your meals ahead of time, you have a strategy. By the time you're ready for your meal, all the chopping, roasting, and other prep work will be done. That means all you have to do is assemble and eat.

Everyone's schedule is different, so figure out a time to prep meals that works for you. For the most part, you will need to carve out about two hours to get all your meal prepping done. Sunday is very popular with my clients, but if Wednesday night is when you have the most free time, by all means do it then. The key is to make meal prep a part of your lifestyle and fit it into your schedule. Like everything in life, the more you do it, the better you get, and the easier it becomes.

Follow the meal prep instructions I detail with each cleanse plan. Having most of your meals ready at the beginning of the week will keep you on track and motivated. Here are some quick tips:

- Make sure you have plenty of airtight containers on hand. I love using glass storage containers that are clear so you can see exactly what is in each one.

- Wash and chop your veggies as soon as you get home from the grocery store. It will only take 15 to 20 minutes and will make such a time-saving difference when cooking throughout the week.

- Cooking in bulk (aka batch cooking) is the most efficient way to use your time in the kitchen. Roast your proteins and vegetables in a large batch at the same time and store in the refrigerator to use later.

- Make any soups, sauces, and dressings ahead of time for use during the week.

- Have fun! Turn on some music and prep it out! It really is so satisfying to get organized and know you have done all the groundwork for your upcoming meals.

DIETARY SUPPLEMENTS

Micronutrients (vitamins and minerals) are vital to your body's ability to function at its best and are essential to your health. I have loaded my cleanses with micronutrient-dense organic veggies (chapter six, page 89, is dedicated entirely to vegetables), but depending on your body's needs, you may want to look into supplements as well.

In general, supplements should be personalized and tailored for each individual. However, there are a few standard supplements I recommend to my clients:

- **Magnesium:** Magnesium deficiency can be common on keto, so supplementing is a good idea. Look for a good-quality brand that has no added sugar.

- **Probiotics:** Probiotics are a requirement! Friendly gut-bacteria ensure that your digestive system is happy and healthy. I like to drink a tablespoon of sauerkraut juice or apple cider vinegar each day. I also take a probiotic capsule daily.

- **MCT oil:** MCT stands for medium-chain triglycerides and is primarily extracted from coconut oil. The oil is relatively flavorless, so I often add it to smoothies, lattes, and salad dressings for an extra dose of healthy fats. Adding a regular dose of MCT oil to your diet is a great daily habit.

- **Vitamin D:** Vitamin D is essential for optimal heath and plays a large role in immune system function. The best way to get vitamin D is to expose your skin to sunlight for 20 to 30 minutes a day at least three times a week. But unless you live near the equator, year-round sun exposure is not possible. In this case, vitamin D supplementation is necessary. I recommend getting your vitamin D levels tested and working with a doctor to determine the best supplement dosage for you.

- **Pink Himalayan salt:** Your body needs salt to help regulate blood pressure, pass nutrients through your cells, and extract excess acidity in the body. Pink Himalayan salt is mined from ancient seabeds and contains a plethora of trace minerals and elements. I recommend a teaspoon of pink Himalayan salt a day, but please check with your doctor if you are over 50 or have elevated blood pressure, diabetes, or any other medical condition.

HYDRATION

During these cleanses, you need to drink lots of water! Each day, drink at least ½ ounce for each pound that you weigh as a minimum. Here are some quick hydration tips:

- Always start your day with a large glass of water. To add extra vitamins and minerals to your glass, squeeze some fresh lemon juice or muddled herbs (like mint or basil) into your water.

- If you are exercising and sweating, add even more water to your routine (at least another 24 ounces).

- To keep your electrolytes in balance, sprinkle some pink Himalayan salt into your water. Pink Himalayan salt is a great source of electrolytes and when combined with water results in faster hydration.

CRAVINGS

If you have a craving, it is probably your brain signaling that it needs energy, or that you are dehydrated. First, drink 12 ounces of water, wait 10 minutes, and see if you are still hungry. If you are still hungry, opt for one of the following fat-fueled snacks:

- Cucumbers with Classic Ranch (page 180)

- Celery with almond butter

- Avocado drizzled with extra-virgin olive oil and pink Himalayan salt

- A handful of macadamia nuts

- 1 cup Healing Bone Broth (page 183) mixed with 1 tablespoon coconut/MCT oil

- Vanilla–Cinnamon Fat Bombs (page 171)

- Golden Milk (page 170)

DEALING WITH KETO FLU

Keto flu can occur when your body is transitioning its energy source from glucose to ketones. Symptoms can include headaches, nausea, fatigue, irritability, constipation, and soreness. Basically, you'll feel like you have the flu for a few days. But don't worry—it lasts only three to five days. Once you get through this transition phase, you begin to reap all the amazing benefits of being in ketosis.

To combat keto flu or to attempt to avoid it all together:

- Stay hydrated. Drink at least ½ ounce of filtered water for each pound that you weigh. Sprinkle pink Himalayan salt into your water to balance your electrolytes.

- Rest. Get plenty of sleep (aim for seven to nine hours each night) and don't overdo it with physical activity or exercise.

- Up your fats. Increase your intake by adding an extra tablespoon of fat to your meals or snacking on high-fat foods like avocados.

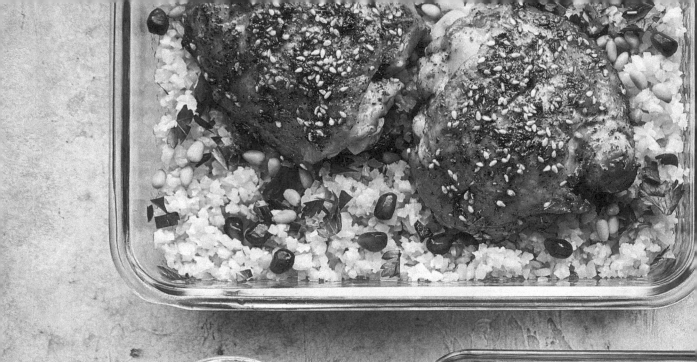

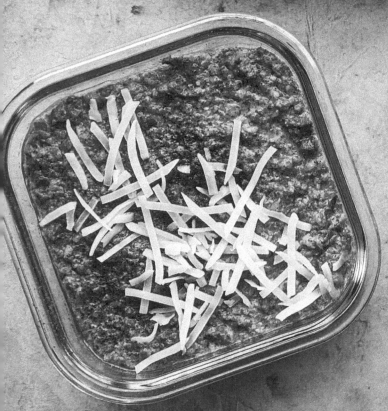

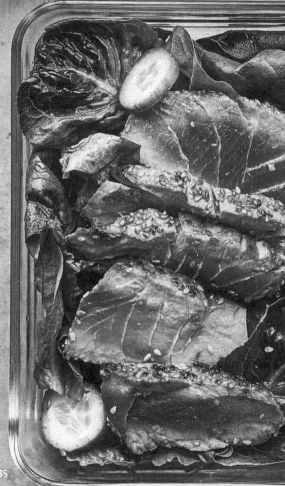

Left: Cinnamon "Noatmeal," page 71
Top: Crispy Lemon–Rosemary Spatchcock Chicken, page 135
Right: Sesame-Crusted Ahi Tuna, 108

CHAPTER THREE

The Cleanses

I know from personal experience that any way of eating only works if you enjoy the foods that you're consuming, the dishes are easy to make, and you feel *satisfied.* In other words, it has to be delicious and satiating—but also practical. So when I set out to create these 14-day keto cleanses, my primary goal was to ensure that the plans met all these attributes.

Each keto cleanse plan includes recipes, shopping lists, and weekend meal prep instructions to ensure that you have all the tools you need to be successful.

Choosing Your Cleanse

The Keto Cleanse: This cleanse is rooted in ketogenic principles and designed to get you into and/or maintaining ketosis, while removing all processed foods, artificial ingredients, chemical additives, grains, gluten, dairy, and sweeteners.

The Elimination Cleanse: This cleanse takes the Keto Cleanse a step further. In this cleanse, two other food categories will be eliminated: nuts/seeds and nightshades. These foods can be problematic for some people, especially for those suffering from an autoimmune disease, IBS, or leaky gut.

The Intermittent Fast Cleanse: This cleanse will be similar to the Keto Cleanse, with the only difference being the eating schedule. This meal plan will utilize the 16:8 method of intermittent fasting. You will have an eating window of 8 hours each day and will be fasting for the other 16 hours.

Notes on the Plans

SERVING GUIDANCE

- The meal plans are designed for one person. Adjust the recipes accordingly if you are cooking for more than one person.

- I will denote on each meal plan if you should double the recipe so that you can have leftovers. The weekly shopping list takes this double batch into account.

- Store your herbs based on their type:

  - Tender herbs such as parsley, cilantro, dill, and mint should be stored in a glass jar filled with 1 inch of water in the refrigerator. Cover the top of the herbs with plastic bag secured with a rubber band.

  - Sturdy herbs such as thyme, rosemary, chives, and sage should be rolled up in damp paper towels, placed in a large zip-top bag, and stored in the refrigerator.

  - Basil should be stored at room temperature.

- Some recipes call for 1 cup of coconut milk (most cans have 1⅔ cups). If a recipe calls for less than 1 can coconut milk, store the remaining milk in a sealed container in the refrigerator for up to five days. Be sure to shake the can vigorously before opening to blend the solids and the water completely.

MAKING SUBSTITUTIONS

- If you don't like certain foods, feel free to swap them out of the recipes for an equivalent macronutrient on the Foods to Eat Freely list on page 12 (e.g., chicken for salmon or broccoli for asparagus). Make sure you adjust the cooking time and recipe instructions accordingly.

STOCKING YOUR PANTRY FOR THE CLEANSES

- For each 14-day cleanse plan that follows, refer to the chart that follows for the pantry items you will need for the week.

	THE KETO CLEANSE		THE ELIMINATION CLEANSE		THE INTERMITTENT FAST CLEANSE	
	WEEK 1	WEEK 2	WEEK 1	WEEK 2	WEEK 1	WEEK 2
HEALTHY FATS						
Avocado oil	√	√	√	√	√	√
Coconut cream						√
Coconut oil						√
Extra-virgin olive oil	√	√	√	√	√	√
Full-fat coconut milk (8 cans)	√	√	√	√	√	√
Ghee					√	
MCT oil	√	√	√	√	√	√
Sesame oil					√	
Unsweetened shredded coconut			√			√
CONDIMENTS/ SAUCES						
Apple cider vinegar	√				√	√
Balsamic vinegar		√	√	√	√	
Capers (1 jar)					√	√
Coconut aminos	√	√	√	√	√	√
Dijon mustard	√	√		√		
Fish sauce					√	√
Gluten-free vanilla extract		√		√		√
Red wine vinegar	√	√	√	√	√	√
Tomato paste (no-sugar-added)		√				√
Tomato sauce (no-sugar-added)	√					
Yellow mustard						√
NUTS/SEEDS						
Pine nuts	√	√			√	
Sesame seeds					√	

	THE KETO CLEANSE		THE ELIMINATION CLEANSE		THE INTERMITTENT FAST CLEANSE	
	WEEK 1	WEEK 2	WEEK 1	WEEK 2	WEEK 1	WEEK 2
NUTS/SEEDS (CONT.)						
Slivered almonds		√				
DRIED SPICES						
Bay leaves		√	√	√		
Black pepper	√	√	√	√	√	√
Cayenne pepper/chili powder		√			√	
Cinnamon	√			√	√	
Cumin					√	
Curry powder		√	√			
Dried dill						√
Garlic powder					√	√
Garam masala		√				
Onion powder					√	√
Oregano	√			√	√	
Smoked paprika		√			√	√
Pink Himalayan salt	√	√	√	√	√	√
Red pepper flakes	√				√	
Turmeric		√	√			√
Za'atar spice		√				
POWDERS/TEAS						
Collagen peptides	√	√		√	√	√
Earl Grey tea bags		√				√
Matcha powder	√			√	√	
Dried lavender (optional)		√				√
OTHER						
Ramekins (oven-safe)						√
Wooden or metal skewers		√		√		

The Keto Cleanse

Welcome to the Keto Cleanse! This plan is great for beginners as well as people who have had success with keto before but may need a reset. All the recipes are grain-free, gluten-free, dairy-free, and sweetener-free.

WEEK 1	MEAL 1	MEAL 2	MEAL 3
MONDAY	Coconut Matcha (page 168)	Kitchen Sink Salad (page 74)	Skirt Steak with Cilantro Sauce (page 151) and Horseradish Cauliflower Mash (page 99) **Double the Skirt Steak recipe**
TUESDAY	Coconut Matcha (page 168)	Leftover Skirt Steak with Cilantro Sauce and Horseradish Cauliflower Mash	Dijon-Glazed Salmon (page 109)
WEDNESDAY	Coconut Matcha (page 168)	Tuna Niçoise Salad (page 77)	Peach-Glazed Chicken Thighs (page 126) and Garlic Spinach with Pine Nuts (page 94) **Double the recipes**
THURSDAY	Coconut Matcha (page 168)	Leftover Peach-Glazed Chicken Thighs and Garlic Spinach with Pine Nuts	Italian Turkey Bolognese (page 140)
FRIDAY	Coconut Matcha (page 168)	Kitchen Sink Salad (page 74)	Skirt Steak with Cilantro Sauce (page 151) and Horseradish Cauliflower Mash (page 99) **Double the Skirt Steak recipe**
SATURDAY	Coconut Matcha (page 168)	Leftover Skirt Steak with Cilantro Sauce and Horseradish Cauliflower Mash	Dijon-Glazed Salmon (page 109)
SUNDAY	Coconut Matcha (page 168)	Tuna Niçoise Salad (page 77)	Italian Turkey Bolognese (page 140)

WEEK 1 SHOPPING LIST

Refer to the Pantry Staples Checklist (page 36) so that you are properly stocked as you go into your two-week cleanse.

FRUITS

- 1 avocado
- 1 lemon
- 5 limes
- 1 peach

VEGGIES

- 12 aspara-gus spears
- 12 cups baby spinach
- 1 cauliflower head
- 8 cherry tomatoes
- 1 cucumber
- 4 cups mixed greens
- 6-8 round red radishes (usually sold in a bunch)
- 1 red onion
- 1 yellow onion
- 1 zucchini

FRESH HERBS AND SPICES

- 3 garlic heads
- 1 (2-inch) piece ginger root
- 1 bunch basil
- 1 bunch cilantro
- 1 bunch parsley
- 2 teaspoons fresh herbs (optional)
- ½ cup pitted Kalamata olives
- 2 tablespoons prepared horseradish

QUALITY PROTEIN

- 2 eggs
- 2 cans tuna (packed in olive oil)
- 4 boneless, skinless chicken thighs
- 4 skin-on chicken thighs
- ¾ pound (12-ounces) ground turkey (dark meat if possible)
- 2 (6-ounce) salmon fillets
- 1½ pounds (24-ounces) skirt steak

WEEK 1 PREP AHEAD

PREPARE THE VEGETABLES

- Chop the cauliflower into florets.
- Peel and dice the cucumber.
- Slice the radishes.
- Peel and dice the yellow onion.
- Peel and halve the red onion. Dice one half and thinly slice the other half.
- Spiralize the zucchini.

COOK AHEAD

- Poach only the four boneless, skinless chicken thighs for the Kitchen Sink Salad (page 74) (you will reserve the four skin-on chicken thighs for use later in the week). Place the chicken in a medium saucepan and add just enough filtered water to cover the chicken completely. Put a lid on your saucepan and bring to a simmer over medium heat. As soon as the water reaches a simmer, reduce the heat to low and cook the chicken for 10 to 15 minutes, or until fully cooked through. Remove the chicken thighs from the water and let cool before shredding with two forks.

- Make a double batch of the Horseradish Cauliflower Mash (page 99), which will yield four servings. Store it in the refrigerator in a sealed container to eat during the week.

- Prepare the marinade for two servings of the Skirt Steak with Cilantro Sauce (page 151). Add your steak to the marinade and store it in a sealed container in the refrigerator overnight. You will make these steaks on Monday night and eat one for dinner and keep one for lunch on Tuesday.

- Make a double batch of the Dijon Vinaigrette (page 178). Store it in the refrigerator in a sealed container for the Kitchen Sink Salad (page 74) and Tuna Niçoise Salad (page 77) you'll eat throughout the week.

- Make four servings of the Cilantro Sauce (page 151). Store it in the refrigerator in a sealed container for the Skirt Steak with Cilantro Sauce (page 151) you'll eat throughout the week.

- Make the two servings of the Bolognese Sauce (page 140). Store it in the refrigerator in a sealed container for the Italian Turkey Bolognese Sauce (page 140) you'll eat on Thursday and Sunday.

- At the end of the week on Thursday night, prepare the marinade for two more servings of the Skirt Steak with Cilantro Sauce. Add your steak to the marinade and store it in a sealed container in the refrigerator overnight.

WEEK 2	MEAL 1	MEAL 2	MEAL 3
MONDAY	London Fog Earl Grey Latte (page 167)	Italian Tuscan Soup (page 86)	Butter Chicken (page 136) **Double the recipe**
TUESDAY	London Fog Earl Grey Latte (page 167)	Leftover Butter Chicken	Balsamic Teriyaki Halibut (page 113) and Ginger Bok Choy (page 95)
WEDNESDAY	London Fog Earl Grey Latte (page 167)	Leftover Italian Tuscan Soup	Steak Shish Kebabs (page 145) and Grilled Zucchini with Romesco Sauce (page 96) **Double the Steak Shish Kebab recipe**
THURSDAY	London Fog Earl Grey Latte (page 167)	Leftover Steak Shish Kebabs and Grilled Zucchini with Romesco Sauce	Seared Sea Bass with Tomato Salad (page 114) and Herbed Mushrooms (page 98)
FRIDAY	London Fog Earl Grey Latte (page 167)	Leftover Italian Tuscan Soup	Za'atar Chicken "Couscous" Bowl (page 130)
SATURDAY	London Fog Earl Grey Latte (page 167)	Leftover Za'atar Chicken "Couscous" Bowl	Balsamic Teriyaki Halibut (page 113) and Ginger Bok Choy (page 95)
SUNDAY	London Fog Earl Grey Latte (page 167)	Leftover Italian Tuscan Soup	Seared Sea Bass with Tomato Salad (page 114) and Herbed Mushrooms (page 98)

WEEK 2 SHOPPING LIST

FRUITS

- 2 avocados
- 3 lemons
- 1 teaspoon pomegranate seeds

VEGGIES

- 1 pound baby bok choy
- 1 carrot
- 4 cups cauliflower rice (or 1 cauliflower head)
- 8 cherry tomatoes
- 4 cups cremini mushrooms
- 1 green bell pepper
- 1 bunch Lacinato kale
- 1 red onion
- 1 jar roasted red peppers
- 8 white button mushrooms
- 2 yellow onions
- 1 zucchini

FRESH HERBS AND SPICES

- 3 garlic heads
- 1 bunch basil
- 1 bunch cilantro
- 1 (2-inch) piece ginger root
- 1 bunch parsley
- 1 bunch thyme

QUALITY PROTEIN

- 1 egg
- 4 boneless, skinless chicken thighs
- 4 skin-on chicken thighs
- 1 pound ground beef
- 2 (6-ounce) halibut fillets
- ¾ pound (12-ounces) top sirloin steak
- 2 (6-ounce) black sea bass fillets
- 6 cups beef bone broth (or make your own, page 183)

WEEK 2 PREP AHEAD

PREPARE THE VEGETABLES

- Peel and chop the carrot into ½-inch pieces.

- Cut the green bell pepper into 1-inch pieces.

- Peel and dice the yellow onions.

- Peel and cut the red onion into 1-inch pieces.

COOK AHEAD

- Make the Italian Tuscan Soup (page 86). Let the soup cool enough to transfer it to a sealed container and store in the refrigerator. The recipe makes four servings and you will eat one serving for lunch on Monday, Wednesday, Friday, and Sunday. Don't dice the avocado until you are ready to serve.

- Make the Romesco Sauce (page 96). Store it in the refrigerator in a sealed container for the Grilled Zucchini and Romesco Sauce (page 96) you'll eat this week for dinner on Wednesday and lunch on Thursday.

- On Tuesday night, prepare the marinade for two servings of the Steak Shish Kebabs (page 145). Add your steak to the marinade and store it in a sealed container in the refrigerator overnight. You will make these kebabs on Wednesday night and eat one serving for dinner and keep one for lunch on Thursday.

- On Thursday night, prepare the marinade for the Za'atar Chicken "Couscous" Bowl (page 130). Add your chicken to the marinade and store it in a sealed container in the refrigerator overnight.

The Elimination Cleanse

The Elimination Cleanse is designed for people who are suffering from symptoms such as fatigue, joint pain, brain fog, aches, and digestive issues. Like the Keto Cleanse, all of the meals in this cleanse are grain-free, gluten-free, dairy-free, and sweetener-free, but two additional food categories are eliminated: nuts/seeds and nightshades. By eliminating these food categories for 14 days, you can assess how you are feeling and determine if you should reintroduce them.

WEEK 1	MEAL 1	MEAL 2	MEAL 3
MONDAY	Green Glow Smoothie (page 63)	Detoxifying Chicken Soup (page 81)	Sage-Roasted Turkey (page 138) and Horseradish Cauliflower Mash (page 99) **Double the Sage-Roasted Turkey recipe**
TUESDAY	Green Glow Smoothie (page 63)	Leftover Sage-Roasted Turkey and Horseradish Cauliflower Mash	Salmon Burger (page 120) and Radish Carpaccio (page 100)
WEDNESDAY	Green Glow Smoothie (page 63)	Leftover Detoxifying Chicken Soup	Sheet Pan Chicken and Broccolini (page 134) **Double the recipe**
THURSDAY	Green Glow Smoothie (page 63)	Leftover Sheet Pan Chicken and Broccolini	Pan-Seared Scallops (page 119) and Dijon Asparagus with Chopped Egg (page 93)
FRIDAY	Green Glow Smoothie (page 63)	Leftover Detoxifying Chicken Soup	Pork Chops with Gremolata (page 156) and Horseradish Cauliflower Mash (page 99) **Double the Pork Chops with Gremolata recipe**
SATURDAY	Green Glow Smoothie (page 63)	Leftover Pork Chops with Gremolata and Horseradish Cauliflower Mash	Salmon Burger (page 120) and Radish Carpaccio (page 100)
SUNDAY	Green Glow Smoothie (page 63)	Leftover Detoxifying Chicken Soup	Pan-Seared Scallops (page 119) and Dijon Asparagus with Chopped Egg (page 93)

WEEK 1 SHOPPING LIST

Refer to the Pantry Staples Checklist (page 36) so you are properly stocked as you go into your two-week cleanse.

FRUITS

- 3 avocados
- 3½ cups frozen avocado (or
- buy 3 avocados and freeze them using the
- instructions on page 63)
- 8 lemons

VEGGIES

- 2 cups arugula
- 12 aspara-gus spears
- 7 cups baby spinach
- 4 Bibb lettuce leaves
- 1 bunch (about 12 stalks) broccolini
- 1 carrot
- 1 cauli-flower head
- 2 celery stalks
- 2 cucumbers
- 2 scallions
- 1 yellow onion
- 2 watermelon radishes

FRESH HERBS AND SPICES

- 3 garlic heads
- 1 bunch basil
- 2 bunches cilantro
- 1 bunch mint
- 1 bunch parsley
- 1 bunch sage
- 8 inches of ginger root (ginger root usually comes in 3- to 4-inch pieces, so grab a few so you have a total of 8 inches)
- 2 tablespoons prepared horseradish

QUALITY PROTEIN

- 3 eggs
- 8 boneless, skinless chicken thighs
- 4 skin-on chicken thighs
- 2 (6-ounce) salmon fillets
- 2 (6-ounce) pork chops
- ¾ pound (12-ounces) scallops
- 2 (6-ounce) turkey cutlets
- 6 cups chicken bone broth (or make your own, page 183)

WEEK 1 PREP AHEAD

PREPARE THE VEGETABLES

- Peel and chop the carrot into ½-inch pieces.
- Chop the cauliflower into florets.
- Chop the celery into ½-inch pieces.
- Thinly slice the scallions.
- Peel and dice the yellow onion.
- Thinly slice the watermelon radishes.

COOK AHEAD

- Hard-boil the eggs. Place two eggs in a small saucepan and add cold water to cover the eggs by several inches. On a stovetop over high heat, bring to a gentle boil and boil for 1 minute. Immediately remove the saucepan from heat and let the eggs sit in the hot water for an additional 12 minutes. Drain the eggs and rinse them in cold water to stop the cooking process. Store in a sealed container in the refrigerator. You will use them in the Dijon Asparagus with Chopped Egg (page 93) for dinner on Thursday and Sunday.

- Make the Detoxifying Chicken Soup (page 81). Let the soup cool enough to transfer it to a sealed container and store in the refrigerator. The recipe makes four servings and you will eat one serving for lunch on Monday, Wednesday, Friday, and Sunday. Don't dice the avocado until you are ready to serve.

- Make a double batch of the Horseradish Cauliflower Mash (page 99), which will yield four servings. Store it in the refrigerator in a sealed container to eat throughout the week.

- Make the Green Goddess Dressing (page 182). Store it in the refrigerator in a sealed container for the Radish Carpaccio (page 100) you'll eat during week.

WEEK 2	MEAL 1	MEAL 2	MEAL 3
MONDAY	Roasted Strawberry Smoothie (page 62)	Creamy Cauliflower and Sausage Soup (page 82)	Zucchini Turkey Burgers (page 139) with Caesar Brussels Sprouts (page 91) **Double the recipes**
TUESDAY	Coconut Matcha (page 168)	Leftover Zucchini Turkey Burgers with Caesar Brussels Sprouts	Dijon-Glazed Salmon (page 109)
WEDNESDAY	Leftover Roasted Strawberry Smoothie (page 62)	Leftover Creamy Cauliflower and Sausage Soup	Greek Lamb Meatballs with Mint Sauce (page 154) **Double the recipe**
THURSDAY	Coconut Matcha (page 168)	Leftover Greek Lamb Meatballs with Mint Sauce	Chicken Paillard with Balsamic Arugula (page 125) and Herbed Mushrooms (page 98)
FRIDAY	Roasted Strawberry Smoothie (page 62)	Leftover Creamy Cauliflower and Sausage Soup	Chinese Beef Skewers (page 144) and Ginger Bok Choy (page 95) **Double the recipes**
SATURDAY	Coconut Matcha (page 168)	Leftover Chinese Beef Skewers and Ginger Bok Choy	Dijon-Glazed Salmon (page 109)
SUNDAY	Leftover Roasted Strawberry Smoothie (page 62)	Leftover Creamy Cauliflower and Sausage Soup	Chicken Paillard with Balsamic Arugula (page 125) and Herbed Mushrooms (page 98)

WEEK 2 SHOPPING LIST

FRUITS

- 2 avocados
- 4 lemons
- 2 cups strawberries

VEGGIES

- 2 cups arugula
- 12 asparagus spears
- 1 pound baby bok choy
- 8 Bibb lettuce leaves
- 3 cups Brussels sprouts
- 1 cauliflower head
- 1 cup frozen cauliflower (or purchase another cauliflower head and freeze)
- 4 cups cremini mushrooms
- 2 scallions
- 1 red onion
- 1 yellow onion
- 2 zucchini

FRESH HERBS AND SPICES

- 3 garlic heads
- 2 cups basil leaves
- 1 (4-inch) piece ginger root
- 1 bunch mint
- 1 bunch parsley
- 1 bunch thyme
- ½ cup pitted Kalamata olives

QUALITY PROTEIN

- 2 eggs
- 2 (6-ounce) boneless, skinless chicken breasts
- ¾ pound (12-ounces) ground turkey (dark meat if possible)
- ¾ pound (12-ounces) ground lamb
- 1½ pounds no-sugar-added pork sausage (can also use ground pork)
- 2 (6-ounce) salmon fillets
- ¾ pound (12-ounces) beef sirloin
- 1 tin anchovy fillets (will find these near the canned tuna)
- 6 cups chicken bone broth (or make your own, page 183)

WEEK 2 PREP AHEAD

PREPARE THE VEGETABLES

- Thinly slice the Brussels sprouts.

- Chop the cauliflower into florets.

- Peel and cut the red onion into 1-inch pieces.

- Thinly slice the scallions.

- Trim and halve the strawberries.

- Peel and dice the yellow onion.

- Spiralize one zucchini and grate the other zucchini.

COOK AHEAD

- Make the Creamy Cauliflower and Sausage Soup (page 82). Let the soup cool enough to transfer it to a sealed container and store in the refrigerator. The recipe makes four servings and you will eat one serving for lunch on Monday, Wednesday, Friday, and Sunday. Don't dice the avocado until you are ready to serve.

- Make the Lemon Caesar Dressing (page 179). Store it in the refrigerator in a sealed container for the Caesar Brussels Sprouts (page 91) you'll eat during week.

- Make the Mint Sauce (page 155). Store it in the refrigerator in a sealed container for the Greek Lamb Meatballs and Mint Sauce (page 154) you'll eat during week.

- On Wednesday and Saturday night, prepare the marinade for the Chicken Paillard with Balsamic Arugula (page 125). Add your chicken to the marinade and store it in a sealed container in the refrigerator overnight.

The Intermittent Fasting Cleanse

Intermittent fasting and ketosis paired together can be extremely effective for fat burning. This cleanse is similar to the Keto Cleanse, with the only difference being your eating schedule. This plan utilizes the 16:8 method of intermittent fasting, which requires restricting your daily eating period to 8 hours and fasting for 16 hours.

Due to the compressed eating window, each day will contain only two meals rather than three. Aim to have meal 1 at 10 a.m. or later each day and to finish meal 2 by 6 p.m. (This window can be adjusted depending on what works best for your own schedule.) The rest of the time outside these feeding hours, you will not be eating but you can still consume water, unsweetened herbal tea, and bone broth.

WEEK 1	MEAL 1	MEAL 2
MONDAY	Coconut Matcha (page 168) and Caramelized Onion and Zucchini Frittata (page 66)	Sheet Pan Fajitas (page 152)
TUESDAY	Coconut Matcha (page 168) and Herbed Scrambled Eggs with Avocado (page 64)	Sesame-Crusted Ahi Tuna (page 108) and Szechuan Broccoli (page 101)
WEDNESDAY	Coconut Matcha (page 168) and Leftover Caramelized Onion and Zucchini Frittata (page 66)	Southwest Chopped Salad with Shrimp (page 75)
THURSDAY	Coconut Matcha (page 168) and Herbed Scrambled Eggs with Avocado (page 64)	Chicken Piccata (page 128) and Garlic Spinach with Pine Nuts (page 94)
FRIDAY	Coconut Matcha (page 168) and Leftover Caramelized Onion and Zucchini Frittata (page 66)	Sheet Pan Fajitas (page 152)
SATURDAY	Coconut Matcha (page 168) and Herbed Scrambled Eggs with Avocado (page 64)	Sesame-Crusted Ahi Tuna (page 108) and Leftover Szechuan Broccoli (page 101)
SUNDAY	Coconut Matcha (page 168) and Leftover Caramelized Onion and Zucchini Frittata (page 66)	Southwest Chopped Salad with Shrimp (page 75)

WEEK 1 SHOPPING LIST

Refer to the Pantry Staples Checklist (page 36) so you are properly stocked as you go into your two-week cleanse.

FRUITS

- 4 to 6 avocados
- 1 lemon
- 3 limes

VEGGIES

- 4 cups baby spinach
- 4 cups broccoli (1 large head)
- 8 cherry tomatoes
- 1 cucumber
- 1 poblano pepper
- 1 red bell pepper
- 1 red onion
- 1 romaine hearts head
- 1 yellow onion
- 1 zucchini

FRESH HERBS AND SPICES

- 2 garlic heads
- 1 bunch chives
- 1 (2-inch) piece ginger root
- 1 bunch parsley
- 1 bunch cilantro (optional)

QUALITY PROTEIN

- 16 eggs
- 2 skin-on chicken thighs
- 2 (6-ounce) ahi tuna fillets
- ¾ pound (12-ounces) flank steak
- ¾ pound (12-ounces) shrimp
- 1 pound no-sugar-added pork sausage (can also use ground pork)
- ¼ cup chicken bone broth (or you can make your own on page 183)

WEEK 1 PREP AHEAD

PREPARE THE VEGETABLES

- Chop the broccoli into florets.

- Peel and dice the cucumber.

- Thinly slice the poblano pepper.

- Thinly slice the red bell pepper.

- Peel and halve the red onion. Dice one half and thinly slice the other half.

- Chop the romaine lettuce.

- Peel and thinly slice the yellow onion.

- Slice the zucchini into half-moons.

COOK AHEAD

- Make the Caramelized Onion and Zucchini Frittata (page 66). Let it cool enough to transfer to a sealed container and store in the refrigerator.

- Make the Mexi-Ranch Seasoning Blend (page 181). Store in the pantry in a sealed container for use in the Sheet Pan Fajitas (page 152) and Southwest Chopped Salad with Shrimp (page 75).

- Make the Mexi-Ranch Dressing (page 180). Store it in the refrigerator in a sealed container for the Southwest Chopped Salad with Shrimp (page 75) you'll eat this week.

- Make the Chili-Infused Oil (page 187). Store it in the refrigerator in a sealed container for the Szechuan Broccoli (page 101) you'll eat during the week.

WEEK 2	MEAL 1	MEAL 2
MONDAY	London Fog Earl Grey Latte (page 167) and Smoked Salmon Baked Eggs (page 65)	Taco Zucchini Boats (page 141)
TUESDAY	London Fog Earl Grey Latte (page 167) and Fried Eggs with Sautéed Super Greens (page 68)	Turmeric Coconut Mahi-Mahi (page 112) and Roasted Cauliflower Steak with Avocado-Green Sauce (page 102)
WEDNESDAY	London Fog Earl Grey Latte (page 167) and Smoked Salmon Baked Eggs (page 65)	Deconstructed Burger Salad (page 146)
THURSDAY	London Fog Earl Grey Latte (page 167) and Fried Eggs with Sautéed Super Greens (page 68)	Thai Beef Curry with Coconut Rice (page 148)
FRIDAY	London Fog Earl Grey Latte (page 167) and Smoked Salmon Baked Eggs (page 65)	Leftover Taco Zucchini Boats (page 141)
SATURDAY	London Fog Earl Grey Latte (page 167) and Fried Eggs with Sautéed Super Greens (page 68)	Turmeric Coconut Mahi-Mahi (page 112) and Leftover Roasted Cauliflower Steak with Avocado-Green Sauce (page 102)
SUNDAY	London Fog Earl Grey Latte (page 167) and Smoked Salmon Baked Eggs (page 65)	Deconstructed Burger Salad (page 146)

WEEK 2 SHOPPING LIST

FRUITS

- 1 avocado
- 1 lemon
- 1 lime

VEGGIES

- 6 cup greens (spinach, kale, chard, or collards)
- 1 cauli-flower head
- 8 cherry tomatoes
- 1 red bell pepper
- 1 red onion
- 1 romaine hearts head
- 1 yellow onion
- 1 zucchini

FRESH HERBS AND SPICES

- 2 garlic heads
- 1 bunch fresh dill
- 1 bunch cilantro
- 1 to 2 bunches parsley
- 1 bunch Thai basil (can sub regular basil)
- 1 jar Thai red curry paste
- (look for this in the international aisle)
- 1 jar dill pickles (no-sugar-added)

QUALITY PROTEIN

- 16 eggs
- 1 (6-ounce) beef tenderloin
- ¾ pound (12-ounces) ground beef
- ¾ pound (12-ounces) ground turkey
- 8 ounces smoked salmon
- 2 (6-ounce) mahi-mahi fillets

WEEK 2 PREP AHEAD

PREPARE THE VEGETABLES

- Halve the cauliflower head. Slice one half into cauliflower steaks (see instructions on page 102) and cut the other half into florets. Place the cauliflower florets in a food processor and pulse until the mixture resembles rice.

- Slice the red bell pepper.

- Peel and dice the red onion.

- Chop the romaine lettuce.

- Peel and halve the yellow onion. Dice one half and thinly slice the other half.

COOK AHEAD

- Make the Mexi-Ranch Seasoning Blend (page 181). Store in the pantry in a sealed container for use in the Taco Zucchini Boats (page 141).

- Make the Classic Ranch Dressing (page 180). Store it in the refrigerator in a sealed container for the Deconstructed Burger Salad (page 146) you'll eat this week. Make the Avocado-Green Sauce (page 102). Store it in the refrigerator in a sealed container for the Roasted Cauliflower Steak with Avocado-Green Sauce (page 102) you'll eat on Tuesday and Saturday, respectively. Only roast one of the cauliflower steaks on Tuesday and Saturday, respectively.

- Make the taco meat from Taco Zucchini Boats (page 141). Let it cool enough to transfer to a sealed container and store in the refrigerator for use on Monday and Friday. Only roast 1/2 of the zucchini on Monday and Friday, respectively.

PART TWO

Cleansing Keto Recipes

Part 2 of this book is dedicated entirely to delicious recipes that are both keto-friendly and full of whole, real foods. You won't find anything processed in these recipes, and they are also keto, grain-free, gluten-free, dairy-free, and sweetener-free. I have also added the following labels and tips for your convenience:

- **PREP TIME.** The Super-Quick label identifies any recipe that takes 30 minutes or less of active prep time to prepare.

- **DIETARY LABELS.** You'll see labels for recipes that are vegetarian or "Elimination-friendly" (which means they contain no nuts, seeds, or nightshades).

- **HELPFUL TIPS.** Every recipe features at least one tip calling out ingredient swaps, cooking hacks, and smart shopping suggestions.

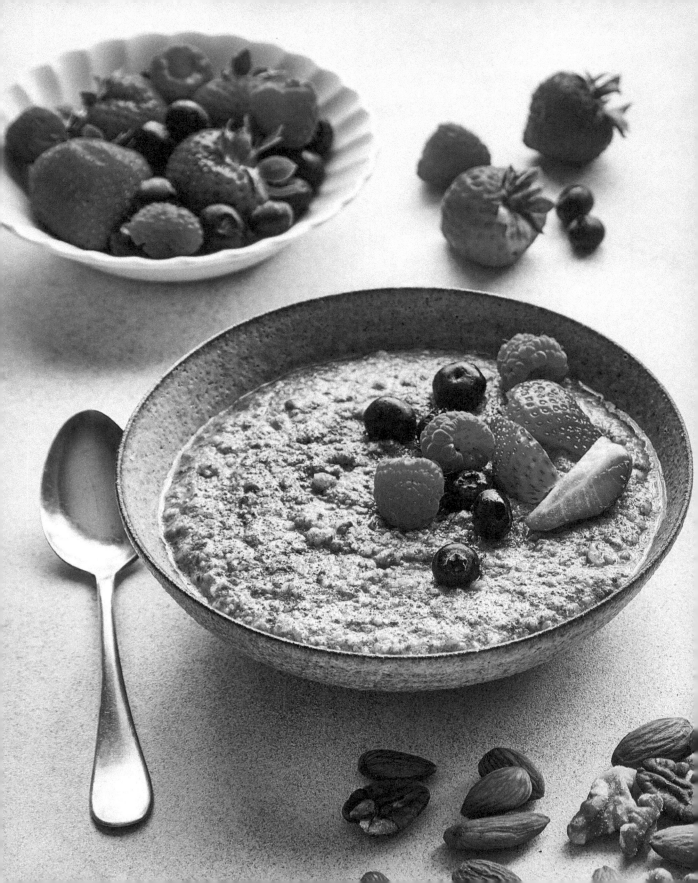

CHAPTER FOUR

Breakfasts and Smoothies

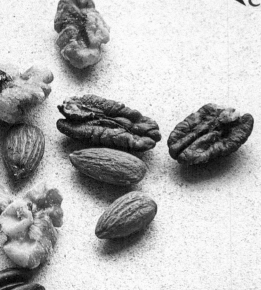

Roasted Strawberry Smoothie

PREP TIME: 10 MINUTES | COOK TIME: 10 MINUTES

Strawberries are the perfect keto-friendly fruit. By roasting them in the oven, the strawberries caramelize and develop a concentrated sweetness as they break down and release their juices, which makes them the perfect smoothie addition. You can also roast the strawberries ahead of time and store them in a sealed container in the refrigerator for up to 3 days.

SUPER-QUICK
ELIMINATION-FRIENDLY
SERVES 2

1 cup strawberries, stemmed and halved

1 teaspoon gluten-free vanilla extract

1½ cups full-fat, unsweetened coconut milk, refrigerated overnight

½ cup frozen cauliflower florets

2 tablespoons collagen peptides

2 teaspoons MCT oil

2 cups ice (plus more, if desired)

1. Preheat the oven to 375°F. Line a baking sheet with parchment paper.

2. In a medium bowl, toss together the strawberries and vanilla.

3. Spread the strawberries in a single layer on the baking sheet and bake for 10 minutes.

4. While the strawberries are roasting, put the coconut milk, cauliflower, collagen peptides, MCT oil, and ice into a blender.

5. Add the roasted strawberries and all the juices from the baking sheet to the blender and process until smooth. Pour into a glass and serve. Store leftovers in a mason jar in the refrigerator for up to 3 days.

TIP I like buying Native Forest Simple Coconut Milk or making my own (page 184). Be sure to shake the container vigorously before opening to combine the coconut and water.

TIP Collagen peptides are sourced from bovine hides or fish scales and are full of amino acids that help support the health of your body's connective tissue, skin, hair, and nails. They have no taste and come in powder form, making them great for smoothies or lattes. My favorite brand is Vital Proteins.

PER SERVING
Calories: 431; Total Fat: 37g; Total Carbs: 11g; Fiber: 2g; Net Carbs: 9g; Protein: 12g
Macronutrients: Fat: 77%; Protein: 11%; Carbs: 12%

Green Glow Smoothie

PREP TIME: 10 MINUTES

Spinach is loaded with vitamins and minerals including iron, magnesium, calcium, folic acid, calcium, vitamins B6 and B9, and antioxidants. Cilantro and cucumbers are known for their detoxifying properties. All three have a mild taste so they don't overpower the flavor of this smoothie, which is fresh and vibrant.

**SUPER-QUICK
ELIMINATION-FRIENDLY
VEGETARIAN
SERVES 1**

1 cup cold, filtered water
1 cup baby spinach
½ cup fresh cilantro, stemmed
1 (1-inch) piece ginger root, peeled
¼ cucumber, juiced
1 lemon, juiced
½ cup frozen avocado
2 tablespoons MCT oil

1. Put the water, spinach, cilantro, ginger root, cucumber, lemon juice, avocado, and MCT oil into a blender and process until smooth.

2. Pour into a glass and serve.

TIP You can find frozen avocado in the freezer section of most grocery stores or you can freeze your own. Wait for your avocados to ripen, then cut them in half, remove the pits, and peel them. Dice the avocado and arrange in one single layer on a parchment paper–lined baking sheet. Transfer the baking sheet to the freezer. Once the avocado cubes are frozen, add them to a sealed container and store in the freezer. You can also use room-temperature avocado, but you'll want to add ice to keep the smoothie sufficiently cold.

PER SERVING
Calories: 410; Total Fat: 38g; Total Carbs: 22g; Fiber: 12g; Net Carbs: 10g; Protein: 6g
Macronutrients: Fat: 83%; Protein: 6%; Carbs: 11%

Herbed Scrambled Eggs with Avocado

PREP TIME: 5 MINUTES | COOK TIME: 5 MINUTES

Most Saturday mornings, you can find me in my kitchen making these scrambled eggs. This dish is the perfect way to use up whatever fresh herbs you have in the refrigerator. I used parsley and chives in this recipe, but feel free to mix and match the herbs to your own liking.

SUPER-QUICK
ELIMINATION-FRIENDLY
VEGETARIAN
SERVES 1

2 eggs
1 teaspoon filtered water
Pink Himalayan salt
2 tablespoons avocado
  oil or ghee
1 tablespoon parsley,
  finely chopped
1 tablespoon chives, finely
  chopped, plus more
  for garnish
1 avocado, sliced

1. Crack the eggs into a bowl, add a teaspoon of filtered water, and whisk them until just combined. Season with salt.

2. Heat a small sauté pan or skillet over medium-high heat. Add the avocado oil and swirl it around the pan for about 1 minute.

3. Add the egg mixture. Use a spatula or wooden spoon to push the eggs toward the center of the pan to form large, soft curds, and cook for about 30 seconds.

4. While the eggs are still slightly runny, remove them from heat. Stir in the parsley and chives.

5. Top the eggs with the avocado slices, a pinch of salt, and a few more chives for garnish.

TIP Feel free to switch up the flavors in this dish by adding smoked salmon, cherry tomatoes, garlic cloves, or shallots.

PER SERVING
Calories: 695; Total Fat: 64g; Total Carbs: 16g; Fiber: 12g; Net Carbs: 4g; Protein: 16g
Macronutrients: Fat: 83%; Protein: 9%; Carbs: 8%

Smoked Salmon Baked Eggs

PREP TIME: 5 MINUTES | **COOK TIME:** 15 MINUTES

This egg dish might look and sound fancy, but it couldn't be easier to make. By topping the eggs with coconut milk before baking them, you will get an extra-creamy texture. This recipe is perfect to serve to a big crowd for a weekend brunch—just increase the ingredients (and ramekins) accordingly.

SUPER-QUICK
ELIMINATION-FRIENDLY
SERVES 1

2 tablespoons avocado oil
2 eggs
Pink Himalayan salt
2 tablespoons full-fat,
  unsweetened coconut
  milk
2 ounces smoked salmon,
  chopped in small strips
1 teaspoon capers
1 teaspoon fresh dill,
  finely chopped

1. Preheat the oven to 375°F and grease the inside of two oven-safe ramekins with the avocado oil.

2. Crack an egg into each ramekin and season with salt. Pour 1 tablespoon of coconut milk over the top of each egg.

3. Bake for 7 to 10 minutes and then set the oven to broil and cook for an additional 1 to 2 minutes. The eggs are ready when the whites are set and the yolks are soft and runny.

4. Let cool for 3 to 5 minutes, then top each egg with an even amount of the smoked salmon, capers, and dill.

TIP I like buying Native Forest Simple Coconut Milk or making my own (page 184). Be sure to shake the container vigorously before opening to combine the coconut and water.

PER SERVING
Calories: 525; Total Fat: 45g; Total Carbs: 2g; Fiber: 0g; Net Carbs: 2g; Protein: 23g
Macronutrients: Fat: 77%; Protein: 18%; Carbs: 5%

Caramelized Onion and Zucchini Frittata

PREP TIME: 15 MINUTES | **COOK TIME:** 30 MINUTES

I am a huge fan of frittatas for their versatility and how easy they are to cook. They have the look and feel of an omelet pie or crustless quiche and the flavor combinations are endless. I love this version that features sweet caramelized onions paired with zucchini and garlic. It is absolutely delicious.

ELIMINATION-FRIENDLY
SERVES 4

4 tablespoons avocado
   oil, divided
1 pound no-sugar-
   added pork sausage or
   ground pork
1 yellow onion, thinly sliced
1 tablespoon
   balsamic vinegar
1 zucchini, cut into
   half-moons
4 garlic cloves, minced
8 large eggs
1 cup full-fat, unsweetened
   coconut milk
Pink Himalayan salt
Freshly ground
   black pepper

1. Preheat the oven to 350°F.

2. Heat 1 tablespoon of avocado oil in an skillet (like a cast iron) over medium-high heat. Add the pork sausage and cook and crumble the meat until it is cooked through and browned, about 8 minutes.

3. Remove the sausage from the skillet with a slotted spoon and place it on a plate, leaving behind the sausage grease.

4. In the same skillet, add 1 tablespoon of avocado oil and the onion slices. Sauté the onion slices for about 6 minutes or until soft. Add the balsamic vinegar to the onions and sauté for another 5 minutes. Remove from the pan and set aside.

5. Add the remaining 2 tablespoons of avocado oil, the zucchini, and garlic cloves to the same skillet and sauté for 5 minutes, or until the zucchini is softened.

6. As the veggies cook, in a small bowl, whisk the eggs and coconut milk until fully combined. Season with salt and pepper.

7. Add the onions back into the skillet and spread them, along with the zucchini, into an even layer. Add the cooked pork over the veggies and pour the egg mixture over top.

8. Use a pot holder to carefully transfer the skillet to the oven and bake for 20 to 30 minutes, or until golden brown on top.

TIP To ensure that the zucchini isn't too watery, halve the zucchini and use a spoon to scrape out the seeds where most of the water is stored and then thinly slice into half-moons. Store any frittata leftovers in a sealed container in the refrigerator for up to 7 days.

TIP I like buying Native Forest Simple Coconut Milk or making my own (page 184). Be sure to shake the container vigorously before opening to combine the coconut and water.

PER SERVING
Calories: 824; Total Fat: 70g; Total Carbs: 9g; Fiber: 1g; Net Carbs: 8g; Protein: 37g
Macronutrients: Fat: 76%; Protein: 18%; Carbs: 6%

Fried Eggs with Sautéed Super Greens

PREP TIME: 5 MINUTES | **COOK TIME:** 20 MINUTES

When it comes to nutrients, leafy greens are powerhouses. They are chock-full of vitamins A, C, and K, plus potassium and fiber. Pair these super greens with fried eggs for the perfect start to your morning.

SUPER-QUICK
ELIMINATION-FRIENDLY
VEGETARIAN
SERVES 1

2 tablespoons avocado
   oil, divided
2 garlic cloves, minced
2 cups greens (spinach,
   kale, chard, or collards),
   coarsely chopped
1 teaspoon apple
   cider vinegar
1 teaspoon pink
   Himalayan salt
2 eggs

1. In a medium sauté pan or skillet, heat 1 tablespoon of avocado oil over medium heat.

2. Add the garlic to the skillet and sauté for 5 minutes. Add the greens and continue to sauté for 10 minutes, or until tender.

3. Turn the heat down to low and stir in the apple cider vinegar and salt. Keep the greens warm in the skillet while you fry up your eggs.

4. In a separate medium skillet, heat the remaining 1 tablespoon of avocado oil over medium heat. Gently tilt the skillet around so the oil fully coats the bottom.

5. Warm the oil until it shimmers, then crack the eggs into the skillet one at a time, being sure to watch out for hot oil splatters!

6. Cook the eggs for 2 to 3 minutes, gently tilting the pan occasionally to redistribute the oil.

7. Transfer the cooked eggs and sautéed greens to a plate.

TIP For deeper flavor (and more healthy fats), pour the excess oil from the fried egg pan over the sautéed greens.

PER SERVING
Calories: 427; Total Fat: 38g; Total Carbs: 5g; Fiber: 1g; Net Carbs: 4g; Protein: 15g
Macronutrients: Fat: 80%; Protein: 14%; Carbs: 6%

Overnight Chia Pudding with Raspberry Compote

PREP TIME: 5 MINUTES | **COOK TIME:** 10 MINUTES, PLUS AT LEAST 2 HOURS COOLING TIME

Overnight chia pudding is a great make-ahead, on-the-go keto breakfast option. I usually make multiple servings at a time in separate mason jars, so they are at-the-ready in the refrigerator. Then all I have to do in the morning is whip up this quick raspberry compote and stir it into the chia pudding for a touch of sweetness. You can swap out raspberries for strawberries, blackberries, or a combination of different berries.

VEGETARIAN

SERVES 1

2 tablespoons chia seeds
1 cup full-fat, unsweetened coconut milk
¼ cup fresh or frozen raspberries
½ teaspoon gluten-free vanilla extract

1. Combine the chia seeds and coconut milk in a mason jar. Put the lid on the jar and shake to combine everything.

2. Once the chia pudding mixture is well combined, put the jar in the refrigerator for at least 2 hours to set.

3. When ready to serve, heat the raspberries and vanilla in a small saucepan over medium heat. Stir continuously until the raspberries are broken down and the juices are at a low simmer, about 5 minutes.

4. Pour the raspberry compote over the chia pudding and stir to combine.

TIP Feel free to double or triple this recipe and make multiple servings in additional mason jars.

TIP I like buying Native Forest Simple Coconut Milk or making my own (page 184). Be sure to shake the container vigorously before opening to combine the coconut and water.

PER SERVING
Calories: 565; Total Fat: 49g; Total Carbs: 20g; Fiber: 12g; Net Carbs: 8g; Protein: 9g
Macronutrients: Fat: 78%; Protein: 6%; Carbs: 16%

Keto Coconut Granola Cereal

PREP TIME: 5 MINUTES | **COOK TIME:** 20 MINUTES, PLUS COOLING TIME

This coconut granola is my keto-friendly version of store-bought cereals that are full of grains and tons of added sugar. The sweetness in this granola comes naturally from coconut rather than from sugar. You will never go back the store-bought stuff after making this recipe.

SUPER-QUICK
VEGETARIAN
SERVES 3
(MAKES 1½ CUPS)

FOR THE GRANOLA

½ cup raw macadamia nuts
½ cup raw sliced almonds
¼ cup cacao nibs
2 tablespoons unsweetened
   shredded coconut
1 teaspoon gluten-free
   vanilla extract
1 teaspoon ground
   cinnamon
¼ teaspoon pink
   Himalayan salt
2 tablespoons coconut
   oil, melted

FOR THE CEREAL

1 cup full-fat, unsweetened
   coconut milk,
   refrigerated overnight

1. Preheat the oven to 325°F. Line a baking sheet with parchment paper.

2. Roughly chop the macadamia nuts into smaller pieces.

3. Into a medium bowl, place the macadamia nuts, almond slices, cacao nibs, shredded coconut, vanilla, cinnamon, and salt and mix with the melted coconut oil.

4. Pour the nut mixture onto the baking sheet and spread out into an even layer.

5. Bake for 15 to 20 minutes, or just until it is fragrant and toasted on the bottom. The mixture can burn easily, so keep an eye on it and stir frequently.

6. Let it cool completely.

7. To serve, transfer ½ cup of granola to a bowl and serve with the coconut milk.

TIP I recommend doubling or tripling this recipe to have it on hand all week. Store leftover granola in a sealed container for 7 days.

TIP I like buying Native Forest Simple Coconut Milk or making my own (page 184). Be sure to shake the container vigorously before opening to combine the coconut and water.

PER SERVING (½ CUP GRANOLA PLUS 1 CUP COCONUT MILK)
Calories: 835; Total Fat: 83g; Total Carbs: 18g; Fiber: 8g; Net Carbs: 10g; Protein: 10g
Macronutrients: Fat: 89%; Protein: 5%; Carbs: 6%

Cinnamon "Noatmeal"

PREP TIME: 5 MINUTES | **COOK TIME:** 5 MINUTES

My version of "noatmeal" (aka keto oatmeal) makes for a healthy, quick breakfast that is also warm and hearty. The cinnamon and coconut make a delicious combination giving this dish the perfect hint of sweetness.

SUPER-QUICK
VEGETARIAN
SERVES 1

¼ cup raw almonds

¼ cup raw pecans

¼ cup raw walnuts

½ cup full-fat unsweetened
  coconut milk

1 teaspoon ground
  cinnamon, plus extra
  for garnish

¼ teaspoon pink
  Himalayan salt

1 tablespoon coconut oil

1. Process the almonds, pecans, and walnuts in a food processor until finely ground.

2. Heat the coconut milk in a small saucepan on medium heat until it begins to simmer.

3. Turn the heat down to low. Add the ground nuts, cinnamon, and salt, stir to combine, and let thicken for 5 minutes. Remove from the heat.

4. Stir in the coconut oil, sprinkle with some extra cinnamon, and serve hot.

TIP Feel free to top this "Noatmeal" with shredded coconut, a few berries, or a dollop of almond butter.

TIP I like buying Native Forest Simple Coconut Milk or making my own (page 184). Be sure to shake the container vigorously before opening to combine the coconut and water.

PER SERVING
Calories: 890; Total Fat: 88g; Total Carbs: 13g; Fiber: 9g; Net Carbs: 4g; Protein: 15g
Macronutrients: Fat: 89%; Protein: 7%; Carbs: 4%

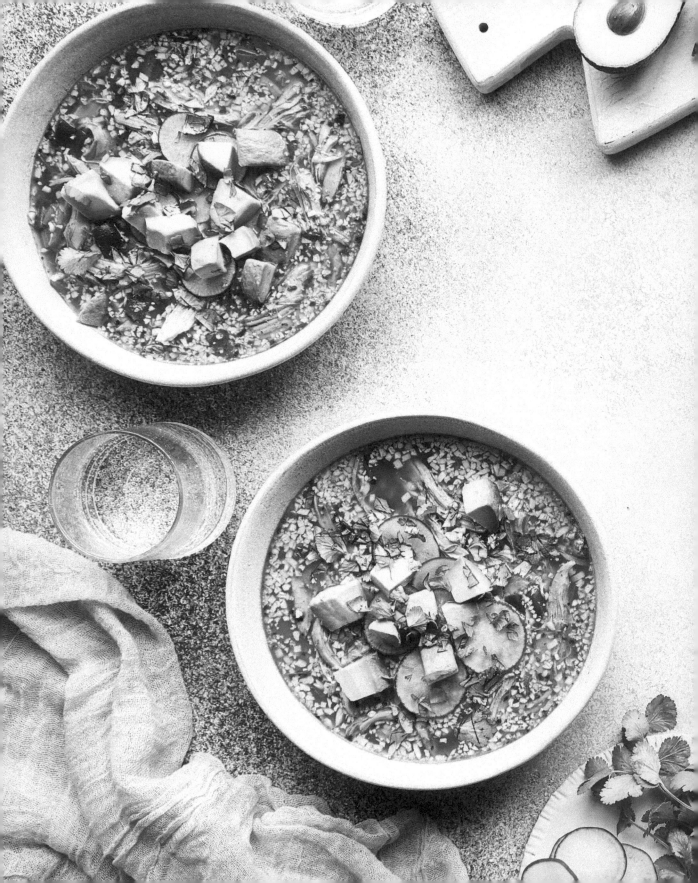

CHAPTER FIVE

Soups and Salads

Kitchen Sink Salad

PREP TIME: 10 MINUTES | **COOK TIME:** 15 MINUTES

The name of this salad comes from the popular phrase, "Everything but the kitchen sink." I have loaded this salad up with tons of colorful, keto-friendly veggies that pack both a nutritional and flavor punch. This recipe also features my simple Dijon vinaigrette, which will soon become your go-to dressing.

SUPER-QUICK
ELIMINATION-FRIENDLY
SERVES 1

2 boneless, skinless
  chicken thighs
2 cups baby spinach
¼ cup cucumber, peeled
  and diced
3 to 4 round red
  radishes, sliced
1 tablespoon thinly sliced
  red onion
½ avocado, diced
¼ cup Dijon Vinaigrette
  (page 178)
1 teaspoon of fresh herbs,
  chopped (optional)

1. In a medium saucepan, place the chicken thighs and add just enough filtered water to cover them completely.

2. Cover the saucepan and bring to a simmer over medium heat. As soon as the water reaches a simmer, reduce the heat to low and cook the chicken for 10 to 15 minutes, or until fully cooked through.

3. Remove the chicken thighs from the water and let cool before shredding with two forks.

4. Place the spinach in a medium bowl.

5. Top with the shredded chicken, cucumbers, radishes, red onion, and avocado.

6. Drizzle the Dijon vinaigrette onto the salad, toss to fully combine, and garnish with fresh herbs (if using).

TIP You can make the shredded chicken ahead of time and store in a sealed container in the refrigerator.

PER SERVING
Calories: 682; Total Fat: 54g; Total Carbs: 14g; Fiber: 9g; Net Carbs: 5g; Protein: 36g
Macronutrients: Fat: 71%; Protein: 21%; Carbs: 8%

Southwest Chopped Salad with Shrimp

PREP TIME: 5 MINUTES | **COOK TIME:** 5 MINUTES

I love a good chopped salad. There is something so satisfying about all the bites being perfectly portioned and the similar size. This particular chopped salad has a Southwestern flair thanks to my homemade Mexi-Ranch Dressing and perfectly seasoned sautéed shrimp. It is so good!

SUPER-QUICK
NUT- AND SEED-FREE
SERVES 1

1 tablespoon avocado oil
6 ounces shrimp, peeled
  and deveined
1 teaspoon ghee
2 teaspoons Mexi-Ranch
  Seasoning Blend
  (page 181)
2 cups romaine
  lettuce, chopped
¼ cup cucumber, peeled
  and diced
1 tablespoon diced
  red onion
½ avocado, diced
4 cherry tomatoes, halved
¼ cup Mexi-Ranch Dressing
  (page 180)

1. In a medium sauté pan or skillet, heat the avocado oil over medium heat.

2. Add the shrimp to the skillet and cook for 2 to 3 minutes per side. Make sure not to overcook them.

3. Use a slotted spoon to transfer the shrimp to a bowl. Add the ghee and seasoning and stir until the shrimp are fully coated.

4. In a medium bowl, place the romaine, cucumbers, red onion, avocado, and cherry tomatoes.

5. Top with the dressing and toss to fully combine. Place the seasoned shrimp on top of the salad.

TIP I love the crunch of crisp romaine lettuce in this salad, but you can definitely swap it out for whatever greens you have on hand.

PER SERVING
Calories: 1,254; Total Fat: 113g; Total Carbs: 23g; Fiber: 10g; Net Carbs: 13g; Protein: 36g
Macronutrients: Fat: 81%; Protein: 11%; Carbs: 8%

Greek Steak Salad

PREP TIME: 5 MINUTES | **COOK TIME:** 15 MINUTES

This salad has all the classic Greek flavors—cucumber, red onion, tomatoes, and oregano. I took the salad up a notch with one of the most flavorful meats that you can cook: steak! Simply dress the salad with lemon juice and extra-virgin olive oil to allow all the flavors to shine.

NUT- AND SEED-FREE
SUPER-QUICK
SERVES 1

2 tablespoons avocado oil
Pink Himalayan
  salt, divided
1 (6-ounce) skirt steak
2 cups mixed greens
¼ cup cucumber, peeled
  and diced
1 tablespoon thinly sliced
  red onion
½ avocado, diced
4 cherry tomatoes, halved
¼ cup extra-virgin olive oil
Juice of ½ lemon
2 teaspoons dried oregano
Freshly ground
  black pepper

1. In a medium sauté pan or skillet, heat the avocado oil over high heat.

2. Salt the steak completely and cook the steak to your desired level of doneness: rare (2 to 3 minutes per side), medium-rare (3 to 4 minutes per side), or medium-well (5 to 7 minutes per side).

3. Transfer the steak to a cutting board and let it rest for 10 minutes.

4. Prepare the salad by tossing the mixed greens, diced cucumbers, red onion, avocado, and tomatoes in a bowl with the extra-virgin olive oil, lemon juice, and oregano.

5. Season with salt and pepper to taste.

6. Slice the steak and arrange it on top of the salad. Make sure to slice it against the grain.

TIP Because skirt steak can be a little tough, your best bet is to tenderize it before cooking. To do that, simply place the skirt steak on a cutting board, cover it with plastic wrap, and then pound the heck out of it using a meat tenderizer or the bottom of a heavy skillet. Let it sit at room temperature for 20 minutes before cooking.

PER SERVING
Calories: 1,313; Total Fat: 116g; Total Carbs: 19g; Fiber: 10g; Net Carbs: 9g; Protein: 49g
Macronutrients: Fat: 80%; Protein: 15%; Carbs: 5%

Tuna Niçoise Salad

PREP TIME: 5 MINUTES | **COOK TIME:** 13 MINUTES

Niçoise salad is my ultimate favorite. My version of this salad is easy to prepare, making it a great lunch or dinner option that couldn't be more satisfying. Opt for the oil-packed tuna, which seals in the flavor and is full of healthy fats. You'll want to check the food label to ensure the ingredients list says "olive oil" and not any other variety of oil.

SUPER-QUICK
NUT- AND SEED-FREE
SERVES 1

1 egg
2 cups mixed greens
1 can oil-packed tuna, drained and flaked with a fork
¼ cup cucumber, peeled and diced
¼ cup thinly sliced red onion
¼ cup pitted Kalamata olives
4 cherry tomatoes, halved
¼ cup Dijon Vinaigrette (page 178)

1. Place the egg in a small saucepan and add cold water to cover the egg by several inches. On a stovetop over high heat, bring to a gentle boil and cook for 1 minute. Immediately remove the saucepan from heat and let the egg sit in the hot water for an additional 12 minutes.

2. Drain the egg and rinse it in cold water to stop the cooking process. When cool enough to handle, peel and halve the egg.

3. In a medium bowl, place the mixed greens.

4. Top with the tuna, egg, cucumbers, red onion, olives, and tomatoes.

5. Drizzle the Dijon vinaigrette onto the salad.

TIP You can store hardboiled eggs in the refrigerator for up to 1 week. Keep them unpeeled until ready to serve.

PER SERVING
Calories: 594; Total Fat: 48g; Total Carbs: 14g; Fiber: 4g; Net Carbs: 10g; Protein: 25g
Macronutrients: Fat: 73%; Protein: 17%; Carbs: 10%

Kale Caesar Salad

PREP TIME: 5 MINUTES | **COOK TIME:** 5 MINUTES

Warning: This salad is addicting! The prosciutto gives this salad a nice, salty crunch and the kale pairs beautifully with my Lemon Caesar Dressing. Trust me, this will soon be in regular rotation each week.

SUPER-QUICK
ELIMINATION-FRIENDLY
SERVES 2

4 to 6 prosciutto slices
1 bunch kale, de-stemmed
  and chopped
2 hardboiled eggs, chopped
½ cup Lemon Caesar
  Dressing (page 179)
Pink Himalayan salt
Freshly ground
  black pepper

1. In a large sauté pan or skillet, panfry the prosciutto slices over medium heat for about 5 minutes (flipping halfway). Transfer the slices to a paper towel–lined plate and set aside. Let cool and then crumble into small pieces.

2. In a large bowl, place the kale, eggs, and prosciutto. Pour in the dressing and toss well. Season with salt and pepper.

TIP This salad is best eaten immediately. If you want to make extras for leftovers, chop your kale, hard-boil your eggs, and make your dressing. Store them in separate sealed containers in the refrigerator. Make the prosciutto and assemble the salad right before you are ready to serve.

PER SERVING
Calories: 646; Total Fat: 55g; Total Carbs: 16g; Fiber: 4g; Net Carbs: 12g; Protein: 21g
Macronutrients: Fat: 77%; Protein: 13%; Carbs: 10%

Sesame Salmon Salad

PREP TIME: 5 MINUTES | COOK TIME: 10 MINUTES

I am always looking to "ketofy" traditional carb-filled dishes, so when I came across a soba noodle salad at my local deli, I made it my mission to come up with an upgraded version. I used spiralized cucumbers as my noodles and then loaded it up with traditional Asian flavors to give it the same amazing taste.

SUPER-QUICK

SERVES 1

FOR THE SALAD

1 (6-ounce) skin-on
   salmon fillet
Pink Himalayan salt
2 teaspoons
   coconut aminos
1 radish, thinly sliced
½ cucumber, spiralized
½ avocado, diced
1 scallion, thinly sliced
1 tablespoon sesame seeds
   (optional)

**FOR THE LIME TAHINI
DRESSING**

1/4 cup filtered water
1 tablespoon tahini
1 tablespoon cilantro
   leaves, stemmed
1 teaspoon lime juice,
   freshly squeezed
1 teaspoon coconut aminos
Pink Himalayan salt
   to taste

1. Pat the salmon dry, then sprinkle the skin side with salt (this will help absorb the excess moisture from the skin).

2. Heat a medium sauté pan or skillet over medium heat.

3. Place the salmon skin-side down in the skillet. Cook for about 6 minutes.

4. Reduce the heat and pour the coconut aminos over the salmon.

5. Flip the salmon carefully and cook for 1 to 2 more minutes.

6. While the salmon is cooking, make your lime tahini dressing by placing all the ingredients in a food processor or blender and processing until fully combined and smooth.

7. In a medium bowl, place the radish, cucumber, avocado, and scallions.

8. Pour in the dressing and toss to fully combine. Place the salmon fillet on top and sprinkle with sesame seeds (if using).

TIP If you don't have a spiralizer, you can use a veggie peeler to peel the cucumbers into thin ribbons resembling noodles or dice the cucumber into small pieces.

PER SERVING
Calories: 485; Total Fat: 28g; Total Carbs: 19g; Fiber: 9g; Net Carbs: 10g; Protein: 40g
Macronutrients: Fat: 52%; Protein: 33%; Carbs: 15%

Slow Cooker Chicken Pozole Soup

PREP TIME: 5 MINUTES | **COOK TIME:** 6 TO 8 HOURS

Think of this as an upgraded classic chicken soup with fresh veggies, healing bone broth, and Mexican spices. It's so easy to make—just throw the ingredients in the slow cooker and let it simmer all day.

SUPER-QUICK
NUT- AND SEED-FREE
SERVES 4

2 tablespoons avocado oil
1 yellow onion, chopped
2 poblano
  peppers, chopped
2 garlic cloves, minced
6 cups chicken bone broth
  (store-bought or Healing
  Bone Broth, page 183)
4 boneless, skinless
  chicken thighs
1 tablespoon cumin
1 tablespoon oregano
2 teaspoons chili powder
2 teaspoons pink
  Himalayan salt
½ teaspoon freshly ground
  black pepper
2 cups cauliflower rice

FOR THE GARNISH

2 avocados, diced
2 red radishes, sliced
2 tablespoons fresh
  cilantro, chopped

1. In a large sauté pan or skillet, heat the avocado oil over medium heat. Add the onion and peppers and sauté for about 4 minutes, or until soft.

2. Add the garlic and sauté for another minute.

3. Transfer the sautéed veggies to a slow cooker and place the bone broth, chicken thighs, cumin, oregano, chili powder, salt, and pepper into the slow cooker. Cook on low for 6 to 8 hours.

4. Remove the chicken and allow it to cool for 5 minutes before shredding it using two forks.

5. Return the shredded chicken to the slow cooker along with the cauliflower rice and cook for another 10 minutes.

6. Transfer the soup to a large bowl and garnish with the avocado, radish, and cilantro before serving.

TIP Find premade cauliflower rice in the produce section or make your own: Buy a whole cauliflower head, chop it into florets, and place the cauliflower florets in a food processor. Pulse until the mixture resembles rice.

PER SERVING
Calories: 454; **Total Fat:** 30g; **Total Carbs:** 17g; **Fiber:** 9g; **Net Carbs:** 8g; **Protein:** 34g
Macronutrients: Fat: 59%; Protein: 30%; Carbs: 11%

Detoxifying Chicken Soup

PREP TIME: 5 MINUTES | COOK TIME: 30 MINUTES

This soup is full of immune-boosting ingredients including ginger, garlic, bone broth—and the powerhouse spice turmeric. Turmeric, and especially its most active compound curcumin, is known to be very anti-inflammatory.

ELIMINATION-FRIENDLY
SERVES 4

4 tablespoons avocado oil
½ cup celery, chopped into ½-inch pieces
½ cup yellow onion, diced
¼ cup carrots, chopped into ½-inch pieces
2 garlic cloves, minced
6 cups chicken bone broth (store-bought or Healing Bone Broth, page 183)
1½ tablespoons fresh parsley, chopped
1 bay leaf
8 boneless, skinless chicken thighs
2 teaspoons turmeric
1 teaspoon curry powder
1 teaspoon grated ginger root
1 teaspoon pink Himalayan salt
2½ cups full-fat, unsweetened coconut milk
2 avocados, diced

1. In a large pot, heat the avocado oil over medium heat. Add the celery, onion, and carrots, and sauté for about 4 minutes, or until soft.

2. Add the garlic and sauté for another minute.

3. Add the bone broth, parsley, bay leaf, turmeric, curry powder, ginger root, salt, and chicken thighs to the pot.

4. Bring to a boil, then cover with a lid and reduce the heat to low and simmer for 10 to 15 minutes, or until the chicken is cooked through.

5. Remove the chicken and allow it to cool for 5 minutes before shredding it using two forks.

6. Whisk the coconut milk into the soup.

7. Return the shredded chicken to the soup and stir to combine. Let it simmer for 5 more minutes.

8. Top with the diced avocado just before serving.

TIP This soup is a great way to use up any vegetables and fresh herbs that have been sitting around, such as zucchini, leeks, rosemary, or thyme.

TIP I like buying Native Forest Simple Coconut Milk or making my own (page 184). Be sure to shake the container vigorously before opening to combine the coconut and water.

PER SERVING
Calories: 891; Total Fat: 70g; Total Carbs: 16g; Fiber: 7g; Net Carbs: 9g; Protein: 50g
Macronutrients: Fat: 71%; Protein: 22%; Carbs: 7%

Creamy Cauliflower and Sausage Soup

PREP TIME: 5 MINUTES | **COOK TIME:** 45 MINUTES

This creamy cauliflower and sausage soup is the perfect option if you are looking for a hearty and filling meal. Make sure to use pork sausage with no added sugars and artificial ingredients or alternatively use ground pork. Both taste great and pair amazingly well with the cauliflower and garlic.

ELIMINATION-FRIENDLY
SERVES 4

1 tablespoon avocado oil

1½ pounds no-sugar-added pork sausage or ground pork

1 yellow onion, diced

4 garlic cloves, minced

6 cups chicken bone broth (store-bought or Healing Bone Broth, page 183)

1 cup full-fat, unsweetened coconut milk

1 cauliflower head, chopped into florets (about 4 cups)

3 thyme sprigs, plus more for garnish

1 bay leaf

1 teaspoon pink Himalayan salt

1. Heat the avocado oil in a large pot over medium-high heat, add the pork sausage, and cook and crumble the meat until it is cooked through and browned, about 8 minutes.

2. Remove the sausage from the pot with a slotted spoon and place on a plate, leaving behind the sausage grease.

3. In the same large pot, add the onion and garlic to cook in the sausage grease and sauté, stirring constantly until onion is softened, about 5 minutes.

4. Add the bone broth, coconut milk, cauliflower, thyme, bay leaf, and salt to the pot.

5. Cover and cook for 30 minutes or until the cauliflower is completely tender.

6. Remove the bay leaf and thyme sprigs. Using an immersion blender, blend the soup until completely smooth. If you don't have an immersion blender, carefully transfer the soup to a blender in batches and purée.

7. Garnish with the cooked sausage pieces and fresh thyme.

TIP If the soup is too thick, whisk in additional bone broth until you've reached the desired consistency.

TIP I like buying Native Forest Simple Coconut Milk or making my own (page 184). Be sure to shake the container vigorously before opening to combine the coconut and water.

PER SERVING
Calories: 884; Total Fat: 69g; Total Carbs: 14g; Fiber: 4g; Net Carbs: 10g; Protein: 51g
Macronutrients: Fat: 70%; Protein: 23%; Carbs: 7%

Thai Shrimp Soup

PREP TIME: 5 MINUTES | **COOK TIME:** 40 MINUTES

Skip the takeout and make this classic Thai soup at home. It is unbelievably tasty and super simple to make. This coconut milk-based soup is aromatic and flavorful thanks to all the classic Thai ingredients used in the recipe like ginger, red curry, and lime.

NUT- AND SEED-FREE

SERVES 2

1 (1-inch) piece ginger, peeled

4 cups chicken bone broth (store-bought or homemade, page 183)

2 tablespoons lime juice, freshly squeezed

2 tablespoons Thai red curry paste

1 cup white button mushrooms, cut into pieces

1 cup full-fat, unsweetened coconut milk

1 tablespoon fish sauce (like Red Boat brand)

2 tablespoons fresh cilantro, chopped

12 ounces shrimp, peeled and deveined

1 lime, cut into 6 wedges

1. With the back of a knife, lightly smash the ginger. This helps release its oils and flavors, so don't skip this step.

2. In a large pot, bring the ginger, bone broth, lime juice, and red curry paste to a boil, then reduce the heat to low and simmer for 10 minutes.

3. Use a slotted spoon to remove the ginger piece from the soup.

4. Reduce the heat to low and add the mushrooms.

5. Cook for 25 minutes then stir in the coconut milk, fish sauce, cilantro, and shrimp. Cook for 2 to 3 more minutes making sure not to overcook the shrimp.

6. Serve immediately with lime wedges.

TIP Find red curry paste in the international aisle of your grocery store. My favorite brand is Thai Kitchen.

TIP I like buying Native Forest Simple Coconut Milk or making my own (page 184). Be sure to shake the container vigorously before opening to combine the coconut and water.

PER SERVING
Calories: 511; Total Fat: 29g; Total Carbs: 13g; Fiber: 2g; Net Carbs: 11g; Protein: 48g
Macronutrients: Fat: 51%; Protein: 38%; Carbs: 11%

Beef and Vegetable Soup

PREP TIME: 5 MINUTES | **COOK TIME:** 35 MINUTES

This soup is an instant classic. I took old-fashioned beef stew and got rid of all the thickening agents (aka flour) and upped its healing power with bone broth. The stew beef gets more tender the longer it cooks, so the more time you let this soup simmer, the better.

NUT- AND SEED-FREE
SERVES 4

4 tablespoons avocado oil, divided
1½ pounds stew beef
Pink Himalayan salt
Freshly ground black pepper
¼ cup carrots, chopped into ½-inch pieces
½ cup celery, chopped into ½-inch pieces
½ cup yellow onion, diced
2 garlic cloves, minced
6 cups beef bone broth (store-bought or Healing Bone Broth, page 183)
1 (14-ounce) can diced tomatoes
1 tablespoon fresh parsley, chopped
1 teaspoon dried oregano
½ teaspoon dried thyme

1. In a large pot, heat 2 tablespoons of avocado oil over medium heat. Use paper towels to dab the stew beef dry, then season with salt and pepper. In batches, add the beef to the pot and brown on each side, about 4 minutes.

2. Transfer the browned beef to a plate and set aside.

3. In the same large pot, heat the remaining 2 tablespoons of avocado oil over medium heat. Add the carrots, celery, and onion and sauté for about 4 minutes, or until soft.

4. Add the garlic and sauté for another minute.

5. Add the bone broth, tomatoes, parsley, oregano, thyme, and beef to the pot.

6. Bring to a boil, then cover with a lid and reduce the heat to low. Simmer for 30 minutes.

TIP Stew beef is trimmed beef chuck cut into bite-size cubes; you can find it at your butcher counter. This soup is a great way to use up any vegetables and fresh herbs that have been sitting around, such as zucchini, leeks, rosemary, or thyme.

PER SERVING
Calories: 461; Total Fat: 23g; Total Carbs: 12g; Fiber: 2g; Net Carbs: 10g; Protein: 50g
Macronutrients: Fat: 45%; Protein: 43%; Carbs: 12%

Italian Tuscan Soup

PREP TIME: 5 MINUTES | **COOK TIME:** 40 MINUTES

This soup gets an Italian flair from the homemade meatballs that cook beautifully in the soup broth. I also fill this soup with lots of vegetables like onion, carrots, and kale to pump up the vitamin and mineral content. The result is pure soup perfection.

ELIMINATION-FRIENDLY
SERVES 4

FOR THE MEATBALLS

1 pound ground beef
1 egg, beaten
2 garlic cloves, minced
1 tablespoon fresh
 parsley, chopped
1 tablespoon fresh
 basil, chopped
Pink Himalayan salt
Freshly ground
 black pepper
2 tablespoons avocado oil

TO MAKE THE MEATBALLS

1. In a large bowl, add the ground beef, egg, garlic, parsley, and basil. Season with salt and pepper to taste and use your hands to mix until well incorporated.

2. Roll the meat mixture into small balls (about 1½ inches in diameter). You'll get about 20 meatballs.

3. In a large sauté pan or skillet, heat the avocado oil over medium heat. Cook the meatballs for 3 to 4 minutes, or until all sides are brown. Set aside.

FOR THE SOUP

2 tablespoons avocado oil

1 yellow onion, diced

1 large carrot, chopped into
½-inch pieces

2 garlic cloves, minced

6 cups beef bone broth
(store-bought or Healing
Bone Broth, page 183)

1 cup full-fat, unsweetened
coconut milk

2 bay leaves

1 cup de-stemmed and
chopped Lacinato kale

2 avocados, diced

1 tablespoon fresh
parsley, chopped

TO MAKE THE SOUP

1. In a large pot, heat the avocado oil over medium heat. Add the onion, carrots, and garlic and cook until onions are translucent, about 5 minutes.

2. Add the bone broth, coconut milk, bay leaves, and meatballs into the pot. Bring to a boil, turn down the heat, and simmer for 5 minutes.

3. Add the kale and simmer until the meatballs are cooked through, 5 to 7 minutes.

4. Top with diced avocado. Garnish with fresh parsley and season with salt and pepper to taste before serving.

TIP This soup also tastes great with a spoonful of homemade pesto stirred in. See the recipe for my Basil Pesto on page 189.

PER SERVING
Calories: 823; Total Fat: 69g; Total Carbs: 18g; Fiber: 8g; Net Carbs: 10g; Protein: 33g
Macronutrients: Fat: 75%; Protein: 16%; Carbs: 9%

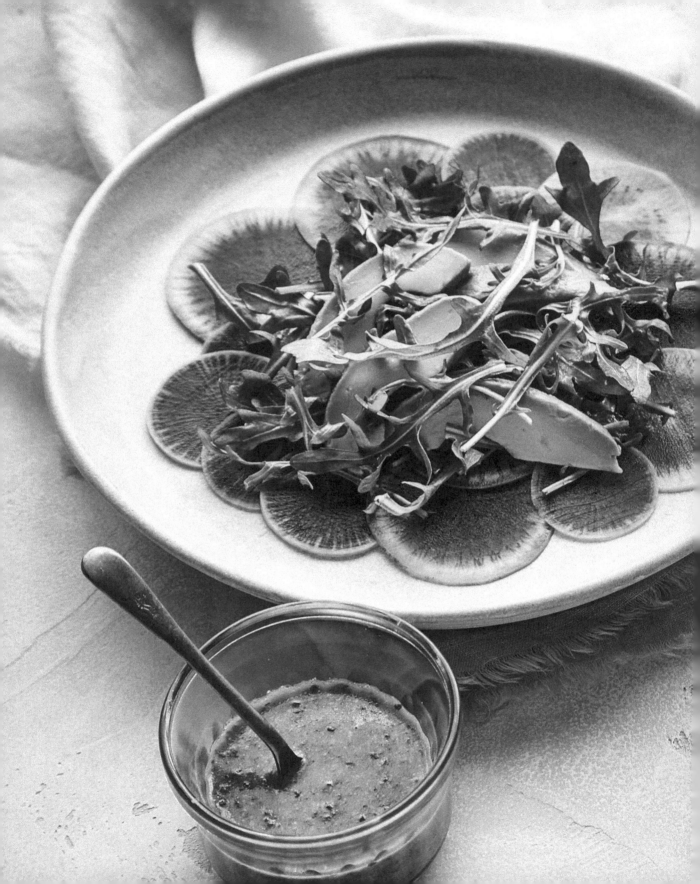

CHAPTER SIX

Vegetables and Side Dishes

Cabbage Slaw with Tahini Dressing

This cabbage slaw is light and refreshing, with the perfect crunchy bite. It is a great make-ahead dish that tastes fantastic with steak, chicken, and seafood. I love to pair it with my Sesame-Crusted Ahi Tuna (page 108) and Coconut-Crusted Chicken (page 124).

SUPER-QUICK
VEGETARIAN
SERVES 1

FOR THE DRESSING

¼ cup fresh cilantro

2 tablespoon filtered water

1 tablespoon tahini

1 tablespoon fresh
   lime juice

1 tablespoon avocado oil

1 garlic clove

FOR THE SLAW

1 cup Napa cabbage,
   thinly sliced

1 cup purple cabbage,
   thinly sliced

1 celery stalk, thinly sliced

¼ red onion, thinly sliced

1 tablespoon cilantro,
   finely chopped

1. To make the tahini dressing, place add all the ingredients in a blender and process until fully incorporated and smooth. Set aside.

2. In a large bowl, combine the Napa cabbage, purple cabbage, celery, red onion, and cilantro.

3. Pour the dressing over the slaw mixture and toss to combine so the slaw is fully coated.

4. Serve chilled or at room temperature.

TIP Store any leftover dressing in a sealed container in the refrigerator for up to 5 days.

PER SERVING
Calories: 288; Total Fat: 23g; Total Carbs: 17g; Fiber: 5g; Net Carbs: 12g; Protein: 6g
Macronutrients: Fat: 72%; Protein: 8%; Carbs: 20%

Caesar Brussels Sprouts

Who knew Brussels sprouts could be such a good lettuce substitute? They give this salad a nice crunch and don't wilt like lettuce does even when covered in my Lemon Caesar Dressing. To complete the dish, garnish with my favorite—avocado!

SUPER-QUICK
ELIMINATION-FRIENDLY
SERVES 1

1½ cups Brussels
  sprouts, trimmed
¼ avocado, diced
¼ cup Lemon Caesar
  Dressing (page 179)

1. Very carefully with a sharp knife, thinly slice the Brussels sprouts. (You can also use a slicing attachment of a food processor.)

2. In a medium bowl, place the Brussels sprouts.

3. Top with the avocado and the Lemon Caesar Dressing and toss to fully combine.

TIP This salad is best eaten immediately. If you want to make extras for leftovers, slice your Brussels sprouts, then make your dressing. Store them in separate sealed containers in the refrigerator. Dice the avocado and assemble the salad right before you are ready to serve.

PER SERVING
Calories: 517; Total Fat: 46g; Total Carbs: 19g; Fiber: 8g; Net Carbs: 11g; Protein: 7g
Macronutrients: Fat: 80%; Protein: 5%; Carbs: 15%

Cilantro–Lime Cauliflower Rice

PREP TIME: 5 MINUTES | **COOK TIME:** 10 MINUTES

Cauliflower makes a perfect substitution for rice and it couldn't be simpler to make. I've added garlic, cilantro, and lime juice to give this side dish a Mexican twist. Use it as a base for a keto taco salad or burrito bowl.

**SUPER-QUICK
ELIMINATION-FRIENDLY
VEGETARIAN
SERVES 3**

¼ cup avocado oil
4 garlic cloves, minced
4 cups cauliflower rice
1 teaspoon pink
  Himalayan salt
Juice of 1 lime
¼ cup fresh
  cilantro, chopped

1. In a large sauté pan or skillet, heat the avocado oil over medium heat.
2. Add the garlic and cook until soft, 3 to 5 minutes.
3. Add the cauliflower rice and stir to combine.
4. Season with salt and cook for about 5 minutes, stirring frequently, or until the cauliflower softens.
5. Remove from the heat and transfer to a serving bowl. Add the lime juice and cilantro and toss gently to combine.

TIP Find premade cauliflower rice in the produce section or make your own: Buy a whole cauliflower head, chop it into florets, and place the cauliflower florets in a food processor. Pulse until the mixture resembles rice.

PER SERVING
Calories: 211; **Total Fat:** 19g; **Total Carbs:** 7g; **Fiber:** 3g; **Net Carbs:** 4g; **Protein:** 3g
Macronutrients: Fat: 81%; Protein: 6%; Carbs: 13%

Dijon Asparagus with Chopped Egg

PREP TIME: 5 MINUTES | **COOK TIME:** 5 MINUTES

I had this dish in Paris and have been in love with it ever since! The flavors are sophisticated, yet so simple. I serve this side dish with my Salmon Skewers (page 111) and Crispy Lemon–Rosemary Spatchcock Chicken (page 135).

SUPER-QUICK
ELIMINATION-FRIENDLY
VEGETARIAN
SERVES 1

1 teaspoon pink
  Himalayan salt
6 asparagus spears, woody
  ends removed
1 hardboiled egg, peeled
2 tablespoons Dijon
  Vinaigrette (page 178)

1. Prepare a large bowl filled with ice water.

2. Fill a large sauté pan or skillet with 1½ inches of filtered water and place over medium-high heat. Add the salt to the water and bring it to a simmer.

3. When the water is simmering, add the asparagus and cook for 2 to 4 minutes.

4. Once the asparagus is cooked through but still firm, place the asparagus in the ice water to keep it from cooking further. Remove the asparagus after 30 seconds and place it on a paper towel–lined plate.

5. Finely chop the hardboiled egg with a knife or use a box grater to grate the egg into small pieces.

6. Transfer the asparagus to a serving dish and top with the Dijon vinaigrette and eggs.

TIP To hard-boil an egg, place the egg in a small saucepan and add cold water to cover the egg by several inches. On a stovetop over high heat, bring to a gentle boil and boil for 1 minute. Immediately remove the saucepan from the heat and let the egg sit in the hot water for an additional 12 minutes. Drain the egg and rinse it in cold water to stop the cooking process.

PER SERVING
Calories: 218; Total Fat: 19g; Total Carbs: 5g; Fiber: 2g; Net Carbs: 3g; Protein: 9g
Macronutrients: Fat: 78%; Protein: 17%; Carbs: 5%

Garlic Spinach with Pine Nuts

PREP TIME: 5 MINUTES | **COOK TIME:** 15 MINUTES

Spinach is hands down a superfood! This leafy green is loaded with tons of nutrients such as iron, magnesium, potassium, and vitamins A and C. I love sautéing spinach with lots of garlic. This recipe uses quite a bit of garlic . . . because well, I am obsessed! Feel free to use fewer cloves of garlic if you aren't as big a fan.

SUPER-QUICK
VEGETARIAN
SERVES 1

1 tablespoon avocado oil

3 garlic cloves, minced

4 cups baby spinach

1 teaspoon apple
   cider vinegar

½ teaspoon pink
   Himalayan salt

1 tablespoon pine
   nuts, toasted

1. In a large sauté pan or skillet, heat the avocado oil over medium heat.

2. Add the garlic and sauté for 5 minutes.

3. Add the spinach and continue to sauté for 10 minutes or until tender.

4. Stir in the apple cider vinegar, salt, and pine nuts.

TIP To toast the pine nuts, place them in a dry skillet over medium-low heat. Cook them for just a few minutes until they are fragrant and golden brown. Stir them constantly to toast them on all sides. When they're golden brown, immediately remove them from the skillet so they don't burn.

PER SERVING
Calories: 241; Total Fat: 20g; Total Carbs: 10g; Fiber: 5g; Net Carbs: 5g; Protein: 6g
Macronutrients: Fat: 75%; Protein: 10%; Carbs: 15%

Ginger Bok Choy

Bok choy is a type of Chinese cabbage and belongs to the cruciferous family of vegetables. It is also an excellent source of folate, potassium, and vitamins K, C, and A. This side dish tastes great with my Chinese Beef Skewers (page 144) and Egg Roll in a Bowl (page 159). If you aren't doing the Elimination Cleanse, I recommend drizzling a teaspoon of Chili-Infused Oil (page 187) over the finished bok choy.

**SUPER-QUICK
ELIMINATION-FRIENDLY
VEGETARIAN
SERVES 1**

2 tablespoons avocado oil

2 garlic cloves, minced

1 teaspoon grated
   ginger root

½ pound baby bok
   choy, halved

2 teaspoons
   coconut aminos

1. In a large sauté pan or skillet, heat the avocado oil over medium heat.

2. Add the garlic and ginger root and sauté for 1 to 2 minutes, or until fragrant.

3. Add the bok choy to the skillet, sauté for 1 minute, and add the coconut aminos.

4. Toss the bok choy and sauté until the leaves are wilted.

5. Immediately remove from the skillet and serve.

TIP Baby bok choy can sometimes harbor dirt within the leaves. To prep the baby bok choy, cut them in half, then rinse with cool water. You can cook the baby bok choy as halves or as individual leaves.

PER SERVING
Calories: 310; Total Fat: 29g; Total Carbs: 9g; Fiber: 2g; Net Carbs: 7g; Protein: 4g
Macronutrients: Fat: 84%; Protein: 5%; Carbs: 11%

Grilled Zucchini with Romesco Sauce

PREP TIME: 5 MINUTES | **COOK TIME:** 5 MINUTES

If you have never tried romesco sauce, get ready to be impressed! This rich, flavorful Spanish dip is made from sliced almonds, roasted red peppers, and tomatoes. It literally tastes good with anything, including grilled veggies, eggs, chicken, and seafood. Make a big batch and use it all week long.

SUPER-QUICK
VEGETARIAN
SERVES 2

**FOR THE
ROMESCO SAUCE**

1 tablespoon avocado oil
¼ cup slivered almonds
1 garlic clove, minced
½ large roasted red pepper
  (from a jar)
2 tablespoons tomato paste
1 tablespoon red
  wine vinegar
¼ teaspoon
  smoked paprika
¼ cup extra-virgin olive oil

1. In a large sauté pan or skillet, heat the avocado oil over medium heat.

2. Add the almonds and garlic and sauté for 1 to 2 minutes, or until fragrant.

3. Transfer the mixture to a food processor and add the roasted red pepper, tomato paste, red wine vinegar, and paprika. Process to combine.

4. Slowly pour in the olive oil and pulse until smooth. Transfer the sauce to a bowl and set aside.

5. Heat your grill or grill pan to high heat.

6. Brush the zucchini on both sides with avocado oil.

7. Grill the zucchini strips for 2 to 3 minutes per side, turning as needed to avoid burning.

FOR THE ZUCCHINI

1 zucchini, cut lengthwise
   into ¼-inch-thick strips
1 tablespoon avocado oil
Pink Himalayan salt
Freshly ground
   black pepper

8. Serve immediately with the romesco sauce. Season
with salt and pepper.

TIP To add a kick to your romesco sauce, feel free to add
¼ teaspoon of cayenne pepper. Start slow and add more
if needed.

TIP Store any leftover sauce in a sealed container in the refrigerator for up to 5 days.

PER SERVING
Calories: 489; **Total Fat:** 48g; **Total Carbs:** 13g; **Fiber:** 4g; **Net Carbs:**
9g; **Protein:** 5g
Macronutrients: Fat: 88%; Protein: 4%; Carbs: 8%

Herbed Mushrooms

PREP TIME: 5 MINUTES | **COOK TIME:** 20 MINUTES

This earthy and herby dish couldn't be easier to make. It is so fast and easy to prepare, you will want to make it again and again. Plus, cremini mushrooms are rich in B vitamins, calcium, iron, selenium, and antioxidants, making them a perfect addition to an anti-inflammatory diet.

SUPER-QUICK
ELIMINATION-FRIENDLY
VEGETARIAN
SERVES 1

1 tablespoon chopped
  fresh thyme
2 garlic cloves, minced
2 tablespoons avocado oil
2 cups whole cremini
  mushrooms, wiped clean
  with a damp towel
1 teaspoon lemon juice
Pink Himalayan salt
Freshly ground
  black pepper

1. Preheat the oven to 375°F. Line a baking sheet with parchment paper.
2. In a large bowl, stir the thyme and garlic into the avocado oil. Add the mushrooms.
3. Spread the mushrooms in a single layer on the baking sheet.
4. Pour the lemon juice over the mushrooms.
5. Sprinkle the mushrooms with salt and pepper.
6. Bake for 15 to 20 minutes, or until browned.

TIP You can substitute sliced white button mushrooms for the cremini mushrooms. You can also sauté the mushrooms in a skillet over medium heat rather than baking them.

PER SERVING
Calories: 315; Total Fat: 29g; Total Carbs: 9g; Fiber: 3g; Net Carbs: 6g; Protein: 7g
Macronutrients: Fat: 83%; Protein: 9%; Carbs: 8%

Horseradish Cauliflower Mash

PREP TIME: 5 MINUTES | COOK TIME: 10 MINUTES

If you've never cooked with horseradish, you must start immediately! Horseradish comes from a root and has a hot, spicy, and peppery taste. It provides so much delicious flavor to this side dish. Pair this with my Seared Sea Bass with Tomato Salad (page 114) and Glazed Lamb Chops (page 153) for a perfect meal.

SUPER-QUICK
ELIMINATION-FRIENDLY
VEGETARIAN
SERVES 2

½ cauliflower head,
   chopped into large florets
   (about 4 cups)
¼ cup extra-virgin olive oil,
   plus more for drizzling
1 tablespoon prepared
   horseradish
Pink Himalayan salt
Freshly ground
   black pepper

1. Fil a large pot with 1 inch of water, insert a steamer basket, and place the cauliflower florets in the basket. Cover with a lid and bring to a boil. Steam for 10 minutes, or until tender.

2. Transfer the steamed cauliflower to a food processor or blender.

3. Add the olive oil and horseradish and process the cauliflower mixture for 2 minutes, or until smooth.

4. Season with salt and pepper to taste and drizzle with additional olive oil.

TIP You can find prepared horseradish in the refrigerated condiment section of your grocery store. The only ingredients on the bottle should be horseradish, vinegar, and salt. If you have never used horseradish or don't like spicy food, start with 1 teaspoon of horseradish, taste, and add more as desired.

PER SERVING
Calories: 292; Total Fat: 28g; Total Carbs: 11g; Fiber: 5g; Net Carbs: 6g; Protein: 4g
Macronutrients: Fat: 86%, Protein: 5%; Carbs: 9%

Radish Carpaccio

PREP TIME: 25 MINUTES

Radishes are crunchy, peppery, and best carpaccio style (i.e., thinly sliced). I use watermelon radishes in this recipe and although they may not look like much from the outside (a boring beige color), when you slice them, they are gorgeously pink inside. This dish tastes great with my Dijon-Glazed Salmon (page 109) and my Peach-Glazed Chicken Thighs (page 126).

SUPER-QUICK
ELIMINATION-FRIENDLY
VEGETARIAN
SERVES 1

1 watermelon radish,
   washed and peeled
Pink Himalayan salt
1 cup arugula
½ avocado, thinly sliced
2 tablespoons Green
   Goddess Dressing
   (page 182)

1. Thinly slice the watermelon radish with a sharp knife or mandoline.

2. Transfer the radish slices to a colander placed in the sink and sprinkle them with salt. Cover and let sit for at least 20 minutes.

3. Drain the radish slices and lightly pat them dry. On a medium plate, arrange them in a single layer.

4. Place a handful of arugula on top of the sliced radishes and top with a few slices of avocado.

5. When ready to serve, drizzle the dressing over the salad.

TIP If you don't have a mandoline slicer, I recommend you get one. They cost about $20 and are perfect for creating uniform veggie slices.

PER SERVING
Calories: 250; Total Fat: 23g; Total Carbs: 10g; Fiber: 7g; Net Carbs: 3g; Protein: 3g
Macronutrients: Fat: 83%; Protein: 5%; Carbs: 12%

Szechuan Broccoli

PREP TIME: 5 MINUTES | **COOK TIME:** 25 MINUTES

This recipe is my "ketofied" version of the popular Chinese takeout dish, but without all the added sugars, starches, or MSG. But don't worry—it is still full of all the spices and flavor. Serve with my Pan-Seared Scallops (page 119) or Salmon Burgers (page 120) and your taste buds will rejoice.

NUT- AND SEED-FREE
SUPER-QUICK
SERVES 2

1 large broccoli head,
 chopped into large florets
 (about 4 cups)
4 garlic cloves, minced
¼ cup avocado oil
Pink Himalayan salt
Freshly ground
 black pepper
1 tablespoon
 coconut aminos
1 tablespoon
 balsamic vinegar
1 teaspoon fish sauce (such
 as Red Boat brand)
1 tablespoon Chili-Infused
 Oil (page 187)

1. Preheat the oven to 375°F. Line a baking sheet with parchment paper.

2. In a medium bowl, toss the broccoli, garlic, and avocado oil together and season with salt and pepper.

3. Spread the broccoli onto the baking sheet in one layer and roast for 20 to 25 minutes.

4. In a small saucepan, heat the coconut aminos, balsamic vinegar, fish sauce, and chili-infused oil over medium heat until bubbling. Reduce the heat to low and let it simmer for 5 minutes.

5. Remove the broccoli from the oven and transfer to a serving dish. Pour the sauce over the broccoli and toss to fully coat.

TIP Don't be afraid of fish sauce! If you haven't used it before, it is a liquid condiment made from fish that has been coated in salt and fermented. It provides incredible umami flavor in many Asian dishes. My favorite brand is Red Boat Fish Sauce. If you don't like spicy food, you can substitute the chili-infused oil for extra-virgin olive oil.

PER SERVING
Calories: 407; Total Fat: 35g; Total Carbs: 13g; Fiber: 4g; Net Carbs: 9g; Protein: 3g
Macronutrients: Fat: 77%; Protein: 3%; Carbs: 10%

Roasted Cauliflower Steak with Avocado-Green Sauce

PREP TIME: 5 MINUTES | **COOK TIME:** 25 MINUTES

Just when you thought cauliflower couldn't do anything more—it can now be *steak*! Just kidding . . . sort of. By cutting your cauliflower into thick slices, you can create a hearty and filling side dish. Don't forget to pair it with the Avocado-Green Sauce; it adds a richness to the roasted cauliflower.

SUPER-QUICK
ELIMINATION-FRIENDLY
VEGETARIAN
SERVES 2

FOR THE CAULIFLOWER

½ cauliflower head
2 tablespoons avocado oil
Pink Himalayan salt
Freshly ground
 black pepper

FOR THE AVOCADO-GREEN SAUCE

2 cups parsley
1 cup cilantro
Juice of 1 lemon
2 garlic cloves
½ avocado
¼ cup extra-virgin olive oil

1. Preheat the oven to 400°F. Line a baking sheet with parchment paper.

2. Remove the leaves from the cauliflower head and then trim off the bottom of the stem, keeping the core intact.

3. With a sharp chef's knife, slice through the middle of the cauliflower head, then cut it into two slices about 1½-inch thick.

4. Place the cauliflower steaks in a single layer on the baking sheet, brush both sides with the avocado oil and season with salt and pepper.

5. Roast for 20 to 25 minutes, or until tender and browned, flipping halfway.

6. In the meantime, make the sauce by placing the parsley, cilantro, lemon juice, garlic, avocado, and olive oil in a food processor or blender and process until fully combined and smooth.

7. Remove the cauliflower steaks from the oven and drizzle with the sauce.

TIP For the Avocado-Green Sauce, feel free to add filtered water to the food processor to get the sauce going and also make sure to scrape down the sides. The end result should be creamy.

TIP This recipe serves two people. If you are planning on just eating one serving, only roast one of the cauliflower "steaks" and store the remaining one in a sealed container in the refrigerator for up to 5 days.

PER SERVING
Calories: 520; Total Fat: 49g; Total Carbs: 20g; Fiber: 10g; Net Carbs: 10g; Protein: 7g
Macronutrients: Fat: 85%; Protein: 5%; Carbs: 10%

Thyme-Roasted Onions

Onions can absolutely be a filling side dish—and this recipe proves it. The key is cooking the onions with plenty of healthy fats. This recipe also adds garlic, thyme, and Dijon mustard for a tangy flavor. These roasted onions are perfect to serve with Mediterranean Basil Pesto Cod (page 116) and Pork Chops with Gremolata (page 156).

ELIMINATION-FRIENDLY
VEGETARIAN
SERVES 4

2 tablespoons lemon juice
2 garlic cloves, minced
1 tablespoon minced fresh
 thyme leaves
1 teaspoon Dijon mustard
½ cup avocado oil
2 red onions, cut into
 1-inch pieces
1 yellow onion, cut into
 1-inch pieces
Pink Himalayan salt
Freshly ground
 black pepper

1. Preheat the oven to 400°F. Line a baking sheet with parchment paper.

2. In a large bowl, combine the lemon juice, garlic, thyme, and Dijon mustard with the avocado oil. Add the onions and toss well.

3. Use a slotted spoon to spread the onions in a single layer on the baking sheet and season with salt and pepper. Reserve the remaining sauce in the bowl.

4. Bake for 30 to 35 minutes, or until browned.

5. Remove the onions from the oven and drizzle the rest of the sauce over top.

TIP The best way to slice the onions is to quarter them, then slice those onion quarters in half. Separate the layers into individual pieces.

PER SERVING
Calories: 297; Total Fat: 28g; Total Carbs: 8g; Fiber: 2g; Net Carbs: 6g; Protein: 1g
Macronutrients: Fat: 85%; Protein: 1%; Carbs: 14%

Basil, Tomato, and Cucumber Salad

PREP TIME: 5 MINUTES | **COOK TIME:** 5 MINUTES

This dish screams summer! There is nothing better than straight-from-the-farm tomatoes and cucumbers paired with fresh basil leaves. I love serving this dish with my Zucchini Turkey Burgers (page 139) and Salmon Skewers (page 111) for the ultimate summer grill-out meal.

SUPER-QUICK
VEGETARIAN
NUT- AND SEED-FREE
SERVES 2

1 ripe heirloom tomato, cut into chunks

8 cherry tomatoes, halved

½ cucumber, peeled and cut into chunks

4 large basil leaves, torn into pieces

¼ cup extra-virgin olive oil

1 tablespoon red wine vinegar

½ teaspoon Pink Himalayan salt

1. In a medium bowl, gently combine the heirloom tomato, cherry tomatoes, cucumber, basil, olive oil, red wine vinegar, and salt. Let the mixture rest for a few minutes to allow the flavors to combine.

2. Taste, and add more salt if needed.

3. Toss again and serve.

TIP Heirloom tomatoes are tomato varieties that have been passed down through several generations of family. They are uniquely shaped and come in various colors: green, yellow, red, and orange. Head to your farmers' market to find the best variety.

PER SERVING
Calories: 278; Total Fat: 28g; Total Carbs: 9g; Fiber: 2g; Net Carbs: 7g; Protein: 2g
Macronutrients: Fat: 91%; Protein: 3%; Carbs: 6%

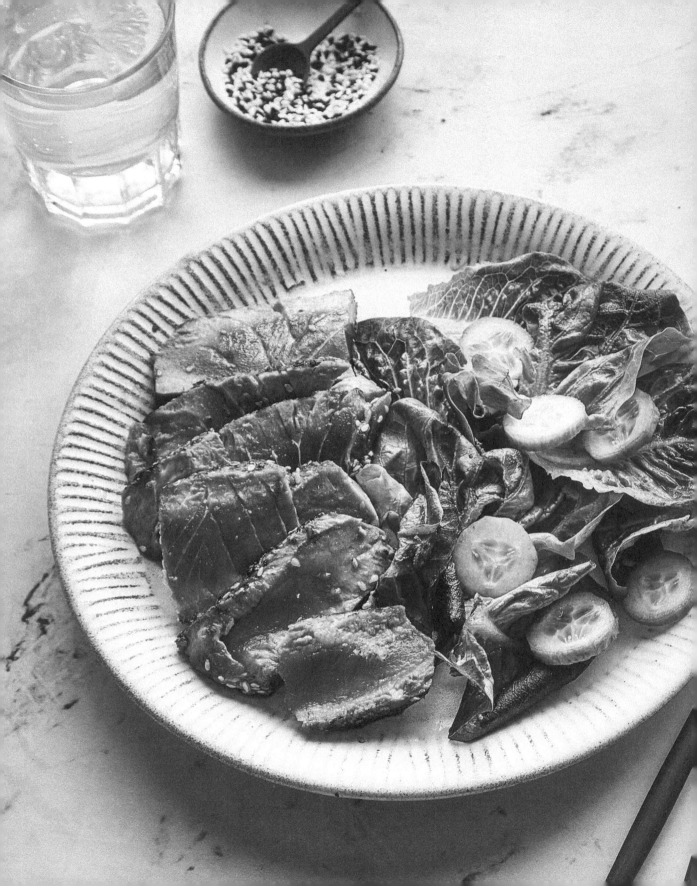

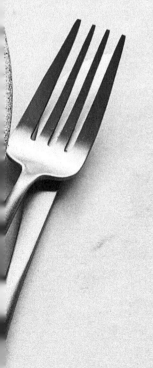

CHAPTER SEVEN

Seafood

Sesame-Crusted Ahi Tuna

PREP TIME: 10 MINUTES, PLUS 10 MINUTES TO OVERNIGHT TO MARINATE | **COOK TIME:** 10 MINUTES

Not only is this dish delicious, but it couldn't be easier to make. You can use white or black sesame seeds for this recipe or even use a combination of both. Serve this tuna on top of a veggie-filled salad or alongside my Cabbage Slaw with Tahini Dressing (page 90) or Ginger Bok Choy (page 95).

SUPER-QUICK

SERVES 1

2 tablespoons
   coconut aminos

1 teaspoon sesame oil

1 teaspoon lime juice

1 garlic clove, minced

1 teaspoon grated
   ginger root

1 (6-ounce) ahi tuna steak

2 tablespoons avocado
   oil, divided

2 tablespoons white
   sesame seeds

1. In a small bowl, combine the coconut aminos, sesame oil, lime juice, garlic, and ginger.

2. Place the tuna steak in a shallow dish and pour the marinade over top. Cover and marinate in the refrigerator for at least 10 minutes, and as long as overnight.

3. Remove the tuna steak from the marinade and pat dry with a paper towel.

4. Fully coat the tuna steak with 1 tablespoon of avocado oil and press the sesame seeds onto all sides of the tuna.

5. Heat the remaining 1 tablespoon of avocado oil in a sauté pan or skillet over high heat. Add the sesame-crusted tuna steak to the skillet and cook for 2 to 3 minutes per side.

TIP This cooking time will result in tuna that is slightly pink in the center. Adjust the cooking depending on how well done you want your tuna. Look for sushi-grade ahi tuna that is fresh and high-quality, especially if you prefer your tuna to be rare.

PER SERVING
Calories: 678; Total Fat: 44g; Total Carbs: 13g; Fiber: 3g; Net Carbs: 10g; Protein: 55g
Macronutrients: Fat: 58%; Protein: 32%; Carbs: 10%

Dijon-Glazed Salmon

PREP TIME: 5 MINUTES | **COOK TIME:** 15 MINUTES

Two words sum up this dish: simple perfection. This complete keto meal takes less than 20 minutes to prepare and is oh-so-satisfying. This recipe will definitely become one of your go-to meals on a busy weeknight.

SUPER-QUICK
ELIMINATION-FRIENDLY
SERVES 1

2 tablespoons avocado
   oil, divided
1 tablespoon Dijon mustard
1 garlic clove, minced
1 teaspoon lemon juice
1 teaspoon fresh parsley,
   finely chopped
1 (6-ounce) salmon fillet
Pink Himalayan salt
Freshly ground
   black pepper
6 asparagus spears, woody
   ends removed

1. Preheat the oven to 425°F. Line a baking sheet with parchment paper.

2. In a small bowl, combine 1 tablespoon of avocado oil, mustard, garlic, lemon juice, and parsley.

3. Place the salmon fillet on the lined baking sheet and season with salt and pepper to taste.

4. Fully coat the top and the sides of the salmon with the mustard mixture.

5. Arrange the asparagus spears around the salmon in a single layer and coat with the remaining 1 tablespoon of avocado oil. Season with salt and pepper.

6. Roast for 12 to 15 minutes, or until the salmon is cooked through to your liking.

TIP Don't have Dijon mustard on hand or don't like the taste? Feel free to omit it from the glaze. The garlic, lemon juice, and parsley still provide incredible flavor to this dish.

PER SERVING
Calories: 481; Total Fat: 34g; Total Carbs: 5g; Fiber: 2g; Net Carbs: 3g; Protein: 35g
Macronutrients: Fat: 64%; Protein: 29%; Carbs: 7%

Salmon Poke Bowl

PREP TIME: 15 MINUTES

In New York City, where I live, there are tons of "make your own" poke bowl restaurants. This recipe was inspired by what I always order at these places: omega-3-rich salmon, lots of low-carb, fiber-rich veggies, and wasabi mayo.

SUPER-QUICK
SERVES 1

FOR THE WASABI MAYO (OPTIONAL)

1 egg, room temperature
2 teaspoons wasabi paste
3 garlic cloves
2 tablespoons lemon juice
1 cup avocado oil

FOR THE BOWL

1 teaspoon coconut aminos
1 teaspoon sesame oil
1 (6-ounce) skinless salmon fillet, cut into cubes
1 cup purple cabbage, shredded
½ cucumber, peeled and diced
½ avocado, diced
1 round red radish, thinly sliced
1 teaspoon sesame seeds
Pink Himalayan salt
Freshly ground black pepper

1. If making the wasabi mayo, place the egg, wasabi, garlic, and lemon juice in the food processor. Process for 30 seconds or so, or until smooth.

2. With the processor running, slowly pour the avocado oil into the food processor until the mixture emulsifies and thickens. Transfer the mayo to a small bowl and store in the refrigerator until ready to use.

3. In a small bowl, combine the coconut aminos and sesame oil. Add the cubed salmon and fully coat.

4. In another bowl, assemble the cabbage, cucumber, avocado, and radish. Place the salmon on top of the veggies and sprinkle with sesame seeds, salt, and pepper. Drizzle the desired amount of wasabi mayo on top.

TIP For the mayo, you can also use wasabi powder and add water to form a paste. The mayo recipe yields 1 cup. Store any leftover mayo in a sealed container in the refrigerator for up to 3 days. This makes a fabulous dip for vegetables and also tastes great as a base for tuna salad.

PER SERVING (WITHOUT OPTIONAL MAYO)
Calories: 423; Total Fat: 26g; Total Carbs: 18g; Fiber: 9g; Net Carbs: 9g; Protein: 37g
Macronutrients: Fat: 55%; Protein: 35%; Carbs: 10%

Salmon Skewers

These skewers are a fun way to cook and serve salmon, especially at a summer cook-out. They are perfect for feeding a large crowd; you just need to adjust the recipe accordingly. Don't forget to make the lemon-caper oil—it provides incredible flavor to the dish, as well as a dose of healthy fats.

SUPER-QUICK
ELIMINATION-FRIENDLY
SERVES 1

FOR THE
SALMON SKEWERS

1 tablespoon avocado oil
2 garlic cloves, minced
1 (6-ounce) skinless salmon
   fillet, cut into 8 cubes
½ lemon, cut into 8 slices
4 skewers (metal, or
   wooden soaked in water
   for 1 hour)
Pink Himalayan salt
Freshly ground
   black pepper

FOR THE
LEMON-CAPER OIL

1 tablespoon capers,
   drained and patted dry
1 tablespoon avocado oil
Juice of ½ lemon

1. Preheat a grill pan over medium heat.

2. In a bowl, combine the avocado oil and minced garlic.

3. Thread the salmon cubes and lemon slices onto two skewers at a time, alternating one by one. Each kebab should have 4 salmon pieces and 4 lemon slices.

4. Brush the garlic mixture onto all sides of the kebabs to fully coat. Season with salt and pepper to taste.

5. Place the kebabs on the grill pan and grill for 10 minutes, making sure to rotate the skewers and cook on all sides.

6. While the kebabs are grilling, in a small bowl, combine the capers and avocado oil. Add the mixture to a small sauté pan or skillet over medium heat.

7. Cook for 2 to 3 minutes, or until the capers are crispy. Transfer the mixture back to the small bowl and stir in the lemon juice.

8. Drizzle the lemon-caper oil over the grilled salmon skewers.

TIP When skewering the lemon slices, fold them in half first. Also, because the salmon is so delicate, use two skewers side by side for each kebab. This will make them sturdier and ensure the salmon doesn't break apart while grilling.

PER SERVING
Calories: 467; Total Fat: 34g; Total Carbs: 10g; Fiber: 3g; Net Carbs: 7g; Protein 34g
Macronutrients: Fat: 66%; Protein: 29%; Carbs: 5%

Turmeric Coconut Mahi-Mahi

PREP TIME: 5 MINUTES | **COOK TIME:** 25 MINUTES

Turmeric and its main active ingredient, curcumin, have powerful anti-inflammatory effects on the body, making it one of my favorite spices to use when cooking. I have paired it with coconut oil and paprika to create a delicious glaze for roasted mahi-mahi.

SUPER-QUICK
NUT- AND SEED-FREE
SERVES 1

1 tablespoon coconut oil
1 teaspoon ground turmeric
½ teaspoon
   smoked paprika
1 (6-ounce) mahi-mahi fillet
Pink Himalayan salt
Freshly ground
   black pepper

1. Preheat the oven to 425°F. Line a baking sheet with parchment paper.
2. In a small bowl, combine the coconut oil, turmeric, and paprika.
3. Place the mahi-mahi on the prepared baking sheet. Season with salt and pepper to taste.
4. Rub the mahi-mahi with the coconut oil mixture and evenly coat.
5. Roast for 20 to 25 minutes, or until the mahi-mahi is cooked through.

TIP Mahi-mahi also tastes great grilled. On a warm summer night, feel free to grill the mahi-mahi for 6 to 8 minutes on each side.

PER SERVING
Calories: 308; Total Fat: 16g; Total Carbs: 2g; Fiber: 1g; Net Carbs: 1g; Protein: 40g
Macronutrients: Fat: 47%; Protein: 52%; Carbs: 1%

Balsamic Teriyaki Halibut

PREP TIME: 5 MINUTES | **COOK TIME:** 15 MINUTES

I have given traditional teriyaki sauce (which contains added sugars) a keto make-over. In my homemade version, I use three simple ingredients to mimic the sweet flavor. This sauce pairs great with halibut, which is a mild white fish.

SUPER-QUICK
ELIMINATION-FRIENDLY
SERVES 1

1 tablespoon
  balsamic vinegar
1 tablespoon
  coconut aminos
1 teaspoon grated
  ginger root
1 tablespoon avocado oil
1 (6-ounce) halibut fillet
Pink Himalayan salt
Freshly ground
  black pepper

1. In a small saucepan, heat the balsamic vinegar, coconut aminos, and grated ginger until it is bubbling. Reduce the heat to low and simmer for 5 minutes. Transfer to a bowl and set aside.

2. In a medium sauté pan or skillet, heat the avocado oil over medium-high heat.

3. Season the halibut with salt and pepper and add the fish to the skillet. Sear for about 3 minutes and then flip and sear the other side for 3 more minutes.

4. Flip once more and brush 1 tablespoon of teriyaki sauce over the top and sides of the fish.

5. Reduce the heat to medium and cook for another 2 minutes on each side, or until the center is opaque.

6. Remove the halibut from the skillet and top with the remaining sauce before serving.

TIP Feel free to substitute cod, sea bass, or salmon for the halibut in this recipe. Also, this teriyaki sauce tastes great drizzled over broccoli, bok choy, and cauliflower rice, so make extra!

PER SERVING
Calories: 393; Total Fat: 19g; Total Carbs: 5g; Fiber: 0g; Net Carbs: 5g; Protein: 45g
Macronutrients: Fat: 44%; Protein: 46%; Carbs: 10%

Seared Sea Bass with Tomato Salad

PREP TIME: 5 MINUTES | **COOK TIME:** 10 MINUTES

This dish reminds me of a warm summer night out east in the Hamptons. The rich, buttery taste of the sea bass pairs perfectly with a fresh, juicy tomato salad. If you have it on hand, I highly recommend adding fresh basil to the salad.

SUPER-QUICK
NUT- AND SEED-FREE
SERVES 1

FOR THE SEA BASS

1 (6-ounce) black sea
   bass fillet
Pink Himalayan salt
Freshly ground
   black pepper
1 tablespoon avocado oil

FOR THE TOMATO SALAD

4 cherry tomatoes, halved
1 tablespoon diced
   red onion
1 tablespoon extra-virgin
   olive oil
½ teaspoon pink
   Himalayan salt

1. Preheat the oven to 375°F.

2. Pat the sea bass dry with a paper towel and season generously with salt and pepper.

3. Heat the avocado oil in a medium-size skillet over high heat until the oil is shimmering.

4. Place the sea bass into the skillet. Sear for 4 minutes on each side, or until the fish is opaque.

5. While the sea bass is cooking, make your tomato salad by combining the tomatoes, red onion, olive oil, and salt in a small bowl.

6. Plate the fish and top it with the tomato salad.

TIP Sea bass is a generic term used for many different types of white fish, some of which are actually a true bass, while others are not. My favorite is black sea bass. You can also substitute another white fish in this recipe if you prefer.

PER SERVING
Calories: 479; Total Fat: 33g; Total Carbs: 4g; Fiber: 1g; Net Carbs: 3g; Protein: 41g
Macronutrients: Fat: 62%; Protein: 34%; Carbs: 4%

Mexican Shrimp Bowl

PREP TIME: 5 MINUTES | **COOK TIME:** 20 MINUTES

I absolutely love roasted shrimp, and this recipe takes it to the next level with classic Mexican spices—and of course garlic. Mix and match your favorite toppings to create the bowl of your dreams!

SUPER-QUICK
NUT- AND SEED-FREE
SERVES 1

¼ red onion, cut into fajita-style strips
¼ red bell pepper, cut into fajita-style strips
2 garlic cloves, minced
2 teaspoons Mexi-Ranch Seasoning (page 181), divided
2 tablespoons avocado oil, divided
6 ounces shrimp, peeled and deveined
1 cup Cilantro–Lime Cauliflower Rice (page 92)
½ avocado, diced (optional)
4 cherry tomatoes, halved (optional)
¼ cup Mexi-Ranch Dressing (optional, page 180)

1. Preheat the oven to 425°F. Line a baking sheet with parchment paper.

2. In a medium bowl, combine the red onion, bell pepper, garlic, 1 teaspoon of seasoning, and 1 tablespoon of avocado oil.

3. Spread the vegetables onto the lined baking sheet and bake for 12 to 15 minutes.

4. Add the shrimp to the same bowl used for the vegetables and mix in the remaining seasoning and avocado oil.

5. Combine to completely coat the shrimp.

6. After 15 minutes, toss the onions and peppers and add the shrimp to the baking sheet and bake for 5 additional minutes, or until the shrimp are pink.

7. Place the cauliflower rice into a bowl, top with the roasted shrimp and vegetables, and garnish with the avocado, tomatoes, and dressing (if using).

TIP If using frozen shrimp, thaw them in the refrigerator overnight. You can also place them in a strainer and run cold tap water over them for 15 minutes or so to defrost them.

PER SERVING
Calories: 635; Total Fat: 50g; Total Carbs: 18g; Fiber: 6g; Net Carbs: 12g; Protein: 32g
Macronutrients: Fat: 71%; Protein: 20%; Carbs: 9%

Mediterranean Basil Pesto Cod

PREP TIME: 5 MINUTES | **COOK TIME:** 20 MINUTES

Baking fish in parchment paper is one of my favorite ways to prepare fish. The parchment paper preserves the tenderness of the fish and also makes for quick cleanup. The basil pesto adds a punch of flavor to this dish, so definitely make a batch for this recipe.

SUPER-QUICK

SERVES 1

1 (6-ounce) cod fillet
1 sheet parchment
   paper, cut into a
   14-by-12-inch piece
1 tablespoon avocado oil
2 tablespoons Basil Pesto
   (page 189)
Pink Himalayan salt
Freshly ground
   black pepper

1. Preheat the oven to 375°F.

2. Place the cod on the sheet of parchment paper and season with salt and pepper.

3. Brush the avocado oil onto the cod and then spoon 1 tablespoon of the basil pesto on top.

4. Close the parchment paper by folding in all four sides to completely enclose the fish.

5. Place the fish packet on a baking sheet and roast for 20 minutes, or until the cod is opaque throughout.

6. Transfer the packet to a plate, open carefully, and spoon the remaining tablespoon of basil pesto on top. Serve.

TIP If you don't have parchment paper, you can still make this recipe, just place the fish directly on the baking sheet.

PER SERVING
Calories: 496; Total Fat: 35g; Total Carbs: 3g; Fiber: 2g; Net Carbs: 1g; Protein: 40g
Macronutrients: Fat: 64%; Protein: 32%; Carbs: 4%

Codfish Sticks with Caper Aioli

PREP TIME: 5 MINUTES | COOK TIME: 15 MINUTES

These aren't your school cafeteria fish sticks. Instead, they are an upgraded version of your childhood favorite using fresh cod and low-carb almond flour to give it a crispy coating. Pair these with a sophisticated and delicious aioli and you have yourself a gourmet meal.

SUPER-QUICK
SERVES 3

FOR THE CAPER AIOLI

1 egg, room temperature
2 tablespoons lemon juice
2 teaspoons capers,
   drained and patted dry
3 garlic cloves
1 cup avocado oil

FOR THE FISH STICKS

1 pound cod
1 egg
1 cup almond flour
1 teaspoon garlic powder
Pink Himalayan salt
Freshly ground
   black pepper

1. Preheat the oven to 425°F. Line a baking sheet with parchment paper.

2. Make the caper aioli. Into the food processor, put the egg, lemon juice, capers, and garlic. Process for 30 seconds or so, until smooth.

3. While still running, slowly pour the avocado oil into the food processor until the mixture emulsifies and thickens. Transfer the mayo to a small bowl and store in the refrigerator until ready to use.

4. Cut the cod horizontally into 1-inch-wide strips.

5. In a shallow dish, beat the egg. In another shallow dish, combine the almond flour and garlic powder. Season with salt and pepper.

6. One at a time, dip each cod strip into the egg mixture and then into the flour mixture to fully coat. Place the "breaded" cod strips in a single layer on the lined baking sheet.

7. Bake for 7 to 8 minutes, then flip the fish sticks over and bake for another 5 minutes.

8. Serve with the caper aioli.

TIP The caper aioli recipe yields 1 cup. Store leftovers in a sealed container in the refrigerator for up to 3 days.

PER SERVING
Calories: 1,124; Total Fat: 98g; Total Carbs: 11g; Fiber: 4g; Net Carbs: 7g; Protein: 46g
Macronutrients: Fat: 78%; Protein: 16%; Carbs: 6%

Cajun Shrimp and Zucchini Noodles

PREP TIME: 10 MINUTES | **COOK TIME:** 5 MINUTES

This quick-and-easy Cajun shrimp recipe requires just a few basic ingredients and only takes 15 minutes to make. The Cajun seasoning gives this dish a spicy, creole feel that contrasts perfectly with the lemony zucchini noodles.

SUPER-QUICK
NUT- AND SEED-FREE
SERVES 1

6 ounces shrimp, peeled
   and deveined
3 tablespoons avocado
   oil, divided
1 garlic clove, minced
1 teaspoon smoked paprika
½ teaspoon garlic powder
½ teaspoon
   cayenne pepper
½ teaspoon onion powder
½ teaspoon dried oregano
½ zucchini, spiralized or
   peeled into noodles
Zest of ½ lemon
Juice of ½ lemon
1 tablespoon chopped
   scallions
Pink Himalayan salt
Freshly ground
   black pepper

1. In a medium bowl, combine the shrimp, 1 tablespoon of avocado oil, garlic, paprika, garlic powder, cayenne, onion powder, and oregano.

2. In a large sauté pan or skillet, heat the remaining 2 tablespoons of avocado oil over medium heat.

3. Add the shrimp mixture, zucchini, lemon zest, lemon juice, and scallions to the skillet.

4. Sauté for 3 to 5 minutes, or until the shrimp are fully cooked, tossing continuously. Season with salt and pepper.

TIP If you don't have a spiralizer, you can buy one online for $20 to $30. Alternatively, you can use a veggie peeler to peel the zucchini lengthwise into thin ribbons resembling noodles.

PER SERVING
Calories: 559; Total Fat: 44g; Total Carbs: 13g; Fiber: 3g; Net Carbs: 10g; Protein: 30g
Macronutrients: Fat: 71%; Protein: 21%; Carbs: 8%

Pan-Seared Scallops

PREP TIME: 5 MINUTES | **COOK TIME:** 5 MINUTES

Scallops are the perfect entrée when you don't have much time to cook. All you have to do is season them with a little salt and pepper and sear them in a skillet for just a few minutes. I love pairing scallops with my Horseradish Cauliflower Mash (page 99) or Szechwan Broccoli (page 101).

SUPER-QUICK
ELIMINATION-FRIENDLY
SERVES 1

1 tablespoon avocado oil
6 ounces scallops,
   rinsed with cold water
   and patted dry with
   paper towel
Pink Himalayan salt
Freshly ground
   black pepper

1. In a sauté pan or skillet, heat the avocado oil over high heat until it begins to smoke.

2. Generously season the scallops with salt and pepper.

3. Gently add the scallops to the skillet, making sure they are not touching.

4. Sear the scallops for 90 seconds, on the top and bottom.

5. The scallops should have a nice golden crust on each side and be translucent in the center.

TIP Make sure to pat the scallops completely dry with a paper towel to absorb as much moisture as you can. This allows the scallops to get a golden crust on each side.

TIP Because scallops cook so quickly, they should be the last item you cook when preparing a meal. Have your side dishes ready to go and as soon as the scallops are done, add them to your plate and serve.

PER SERVING
Calories: 280; Total Fat: 15g; Total Carbs: 4g; Fiber: 0g; Net Carbs: 4g; Protein: 29g
Macronutrients: Fat: 48%; Protein: 41%; Carbs: 11%

Salmon Burger

PREP TIME: 10 MINUTES | **COOK TIME:** 10 MINUTES

If you haven't made salmon burgers before, you must make them ASAP! They are so easy to pull together and this version packs a flavor punch with all the Asian-inspired ingredients. You can easily increase this recipe to feed a large group.

SUPER-QUICK
ELIMINATION-FRIENDLY
SERVES 1

1 (6-ounce) skinless
   salmon fillet, cut into
   1-inch cubes
1 scallion, thinly sliced
1 garlic clove, minced
½ teaspoon fresh
   grated ginger
1 teaspoon coconut aminos
Pink Himalayan salt
Freshly ground
   black pepper
1 tablespoon avocado oil
2 Bibb lettuce leaves

1. Place the salmon cubes in the freezer for about 10 minutes. You want them very cold, but not frozen.

2. Transfer the salmon to a food processor and process for 5 quick 2-second pulses. You don't want the salmon to turn into a paste.

3. Transfer the salmon to a bowl and add the scallion, garlic, ginger, and coconut aminos. Season the mixture with salt and pepper.

4. Use your hands to fully incorporate the ingredients and form into a circular patty about 1-inch thick.

5. In a medium-size skillet, heat the avocado oil over medium-high heat. Add the salmon burger and cook for 3 minutes on each side.

6. Wrap the burger in the Bibb lettuce leaves.

TIP Feel free to top the burger with sliced avocado, radishes, or red onion. This burger also tastes amazing paired with my Wasabi Mayo (page 110).

PER SERVING
Calories: 330; Total Fat: 20g; Total Carbs: 4g; Fiber: 1g; Net Carbs: 3g; Protein: 34g
Macronutrients: Fat: 55%; Protein: 41%; Carbs: 4%

Crab Fried Rice

PREP TIME: 10 MINUTES | **COOK TIME:** 12 MINUTES

Before I was officially keto, crab fried rice was always my dish of choice at Thai restaurants. So I knew I had to come up with a low-carb version that tasted just as good—and I think I nailed it. Full of fresh vegetables, including a cauliflower rice base, this fried rice is as delicious as it is healthy. Look for good-quality lump crabmeat—don't get fooled by imitation crab that comes from pollack.

SUPER-QUICK
SERVES 4

¼ cup avocado oil
½ yellow onion, diced
4 garlic cloves, minced
2 eggs, beaten
6 cups cauliflower rice
¼ cup coconut aminos
1 tablespoon sesame oil
1 (8-ounce) container lump
  crabmeat, drained
8 cherry tomatoes, halved
Pink Himalayan salt
Freshly ground
  black pepper
Chili-Infused Oil (optional,
  page 187)
Fresh chopped cilantro, for
  garnish (optional)
Sliced scallions, for garnish
  (optional)
Sesame seeds, for garnish
  (optional)

1. In a large sauté pan or skillet, heat the avocado oil over medium-high heat. Add the onions and garlic and cook for 3 to 4 minutes, or until soft.

2. Push the onions and garlic to one side of the skillet and pour the eggs into the other side. Let the eggs set for 30 seconds or so.

3. Add the cauliflower rice, coconut aminos, and sesame oil, tossing everything together and breaking up the eggs.

4. Cook the cauliflower rice for about 5 minutes, stirring frequently until the cauliflower softens.

5. Add in the crab and tomatoes and season with salt and pepper. Cook for 2 more minutes and top with chili-infused oil (if using), cilantro, scallions, and sesame seeds.

TIP Find premade cauliflower rice in the produce section or make your own: Buy a whole cauliflower head, chop it into florets, and place the cauliflower florets in a food processor. Pulse until the mixture resembles rice.

TIP For super-crispy rice, transfer the finished product without the optional toppings to an air fryer set to 350°F. Fry for 2 to 3 minutes, toss, and then fry again for another 2 minutes.

PER SERVING
Calories: 302; **Total Fat:** 21g; **Total Carbs:** 13g; **Fiber:** 4g; **Net Carbs:** 9g; **Protein:** 16g
Macronutrients: Fat: 63%; Protein: 21%; Carbs: 16%

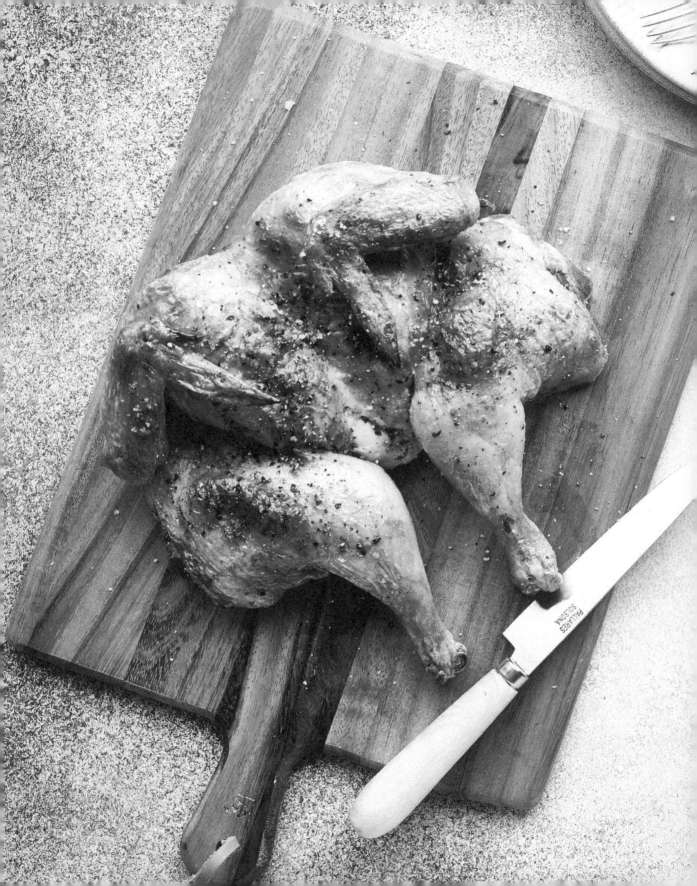

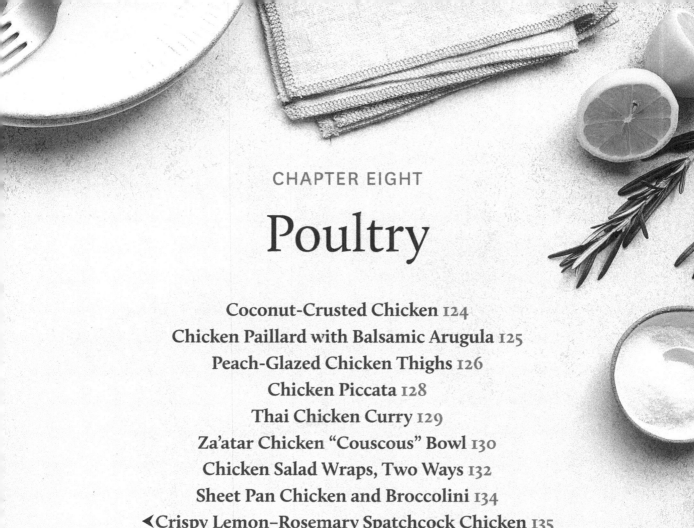

CHAPTER EIGHT

Poultry

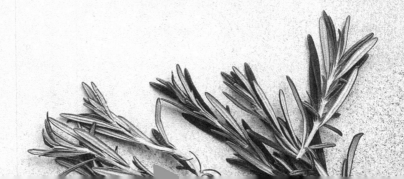

Coconut-Crusted Chicken

PREP TIME: 10 MINUTES | **COOK TIME:** 20 MINUTES

Coconut-crusted chicken is my keto take on the standard chicken tender. I have added a double dose of coconut to this recipe and the end result is a crispy masterpiece that will please both kids and adults. Make a big batch for a quick weeknight family dinner. Note that when you scale up the recipe for four, you'll need only two eggs.

SUPER-QUICK
ELIMINATION-FRIENDLY
SERVES 1

1 egg, beaten
2 tablespoons coconut flour
½ cup unsweetened
   shredded coconut
½ teaspoon garlic powder
3 chicken tenderloins
Pink Himalayan salt
Freshly ground
   black pepper

1. Preheat the oven to 400°F. Line a baking sheet with parchment paper.

2. In one shallow dish, beat the egg. In another shallow dish, put the coconut flour. In a third shallow dish, combine the shredded coconut and garlic powder.

3. Season the chicken tenders with salt and pepper.

4. One at a time, dip each chicken tender into the egg mixture, then into the flour mixture, and then into the shredded coconut mixture to fully coat.

5. Place the "breaded" chicken tenders in a single layer on the lined baking sheet.

6. Bake for 15 to 20 minutes, flipping halfway until they are golden brown and toasted.

TIP You can also make these chicken fingers in the air fryer. Preheat an air fryer to 375°F. Grease the air fryer basket with some avocado oil. Place the chicken tenders in the air fryer basket, making sure they are not touching (fry them in batches if necessary). Cook for 6 minutes, flip the tenders over, and continue cooking for 4 to 6 minutes, or until golden brown.

PER SERVING
Calories: 553; Total Fat: 34g; Total Carbs: 22g; Fiber: 12g; Net Carbs: 10g; Protein: 47g
Macronutrients: Fat: 55%; Protein: 34%; Carbs: 11%

Chicken Paillard with Balsamic Arugula

PREP TIME: 10 MINUTES, PLUS 10 MINUTES TO OVERNIGHT TO MARINATE |
COOK TIME: 10 MINUTES

The word *paillard* is a French cooking term, which means a thinly pounded piece of meat that cooks quickly. By pounding the chicken breast, you not only tenderize it, but also make it much faster to cook—I'm talking 10 minutes. It is a great technique to use when you are looking to get dinner on the table quickly.

SUPER-QUICK
ELIMINATION-FRIENDLY
SERVES 1

1 boneless, skinless
  chicken breast
2 tablespoons avocado
  oil, divided
1 tablespoon red
  wine vinegar
1 tablespoon
  coconut aminos
1 garlic clove, minced
½ teaspoon dried oregano
1 teaspoon
  balsamic vinegar
1 teaspoon extra-virgin
  olive oil
1 cup arugula
Pink Himalayan salt
Freshly ground
  black pepper

1. Wrap the chicken breast in plastic wrap, place it on a cutting board, and use a meat tenderizer (or the bottom of a heavy sauté pan or skillet) to pound it to ¼-inch thick. Set aside.

2. In a small bowl, combine 1 tablespoon of avocado oil, red wine vinegar, coconut aminos, garlic, and oregano.

3. Place the pounded chicken breast in a shallow dish and pour the marinade on top. Cover and marinate in the refrigerator for at least 10 minutes and up to overnight.

4. Heat a skillet over medium-high heat. Add the remaining 2 tablespoons of avocado oil to the pan.

5. Add the chicken to the skillet and cook for 3 minutes. Flip and cook for an additional 5 to 6 minutes.

6. In a small bowl, whisk together the balsamic vinegar and olive oil, and then toss with the arugula. Season with salt and pepper.

7. Transfer the cooked chicken to a plate and top with the dressed arugula.

TIP If you have time, marinate this chicken overnight to allow it to soak up all the incredible flavors of the marinade.

PER SERVING
Calories: 439; Total Fat: 35g; Total Carbs: 6g; Fiber: 1g; Net Carbs: 5g; Protein: 24g
Macronutrients: Fat: 72%; Protein: 22%; Carbs: 6%

Peach-Glazed Chicken Thighs

PREP TIME: 10 MINUTES | **COOK TIME:** 30 MINUTES

Before you ask, yes, you can consume fruit on keto. The trick is to look for lower-carb varieties and to not overdo it. A whole peach has around 12 grams of net carbs, so I recommend sticking with ½ peach as a serving size. A sweet peach makes an incredible glaze for these roasted chicken thighs.

ELIMINATION-FRIENDLY

SERVES 1

2 tablespoons avocado oil

2 skin-on chicken thighs

Pink Himalayan salt

Freshly ground
   black pepper

½ peach, peeled and
   finely diced

¼ cup filtered water

1 teaspoon apple
   cider vinegar

1 teaspoon Dijon mustard

1 teaspoon grated
   ginger root

1. Preheat the oven to 425°F.

2. Heat a skillet over medium-high heat. Pour in the avocado oil and swirl it around to coat.

3. Pat the chicken thighs dry with a paper towel and season with salt and pepper.

4. Add the chicken thighs to the skillet skin-side down. Cook the chicken thighs, without moving them, for 7 to 9 minutes. You want the fat to render so the skin gets nice and crispy.

5. Once the chicken releases from the pan and has a nicely browned crust on the skin, use tongs to flip the chicken thighs over.

6. Carefully transfer the skillet to the oven and roast for 18 to 20 minutes.

7. While the chicken is roasting, in a small saucepan, heat the peach, water, apple cider vinegar, mustard, and grated ginger over medium heat until it is bubbling. Reduce the heat to low and simmer until the chicken is finished cooking.

8. Pour the peach glaze over the chicken thighs and serve.

TIP If peaches are out of season, you can use frozen peaches, but be sure to adjust how much water you need to get the desired consistency.

TIP The easiest way to peel a peach is to make an "x" at the bottom with a sharp knife, and then place it in a pot of boiling water for 15 to 20 seconds. Immediately transfer the peach into an ice-water bath to cool and then use a paring knife to peel the skin.

PER SERVING
Calories: 684; Total Fat: 57g; Total Carbs: 6g; Fiber: 1g; Net Carbs: 5g; Protein: 33g
Macronutrients: Fat: 75%; Protein: 19%; Carbs: 6%

Chicken Piccata

PREP TIME: 5 MINUTES | **COOK TIME:** 25 MINUTES

Chicken piccata is an Italian dish that features the flavors of lemon, capers, and garlic. I have turned this menu staple into a one-pan dish that comes together in just 30 minutes. The end result is amazingly crispy chicken thighs served with a rich lemon sauce. This recipe is a must!

SUPER-QUICK
ELIMINATION-FRIENDLY
SERVES 1

1 tablespoon avocado oil
2 skin-on chicken thighs
Pink Himalayan salt
Freshly ground
    black pepper
2 tablespoons chicken
    bone broth (store-bought
    or Healing Bone Broth,
    page 183)
1 tablespoon ghee
1 tablespoon
    capers, drained
2 garlic cloves, minced
Juice of ½ lemon
½ lemon, sliced

1. Heat a medium skillet over medium-high heat. Add the avocado oil to the pan and swirl it around to coat it.

2. Pat the chicken thighs dry with a paper towel and season with salt and pepper.

3. Add the chicken thighs to the skillet skin-side down. Cook the thighs, without moving them, for 7 to 9 minutes. You want the fat to render so the skin gets nice and crispy.

4. Once the chicken releases from the pan and has a nicely browned crust on the skin, use tongs to flip the chicken thighs over and cook on the other side for 7 to 9 more minutes.

5. Carefully transfer the chicken to a plate and discard the chicken juice from the skillet.

6. Add the bone broth, ghee, capers, garlic, and lemon juice to the skillet. Lower the heat to medium-low and bring it to a simmer.

7. Return the chicken thighs back to the skillet, surround the chicken with the lemon slices, and simmer in the sauce for 5 minutes.

TIP Be careful when searing the chicken thighs in the oil, as there will be splatter. If you have a splatter guard, use it.

PER SERVING
Calories: 555; **Total Fat:** 43g; **Total Carbs:** 7g; **Fiber:** 1g; **Net Carbs:** 6g; **Protein:** 34g
Macronutrients: Fat: 70%; Protein: 25%; Carbs: 5%

Thai Chicken Curry

PREP TIME: 10 MINUTES | **COOK TIME:** 20 MINUTES

Bring on the spice! This Thai chicken curry has such an incredible flavor profile and rivals any takeout curry you would order on your way home from work. This recipe serves one person, but can easily be doubled or tripled to ensure that you have leftovers.

SUPER-QUICK
NUT- AND SEED-FREE
SERVES 1

1 tablespoon coconut oil
¼ yellow onion, diced
2 boneless, skinless
chicken thighs, diced into
1-inch pieces
2 garlic cloves, minced
1 teaspoon grated
ginger root
1 cup full-fat, unsweetened
coconut milk
1 tablespoon Thai red
curry paste
Pink Himalayan salt
Freshly ground
black pepper
1 cup fresh spinach leaves
1 teaspoon lime juice
1 cup Cilantro–Lime
Cauliflower Rice
(page 92)
¼ cup fresh cilantro, finely
chopped (optional)

1. In a medium sauté pan or skillet, heat the coconut oil over medium-high heat. Add the onion and sauté for 3 to 4 minutes, until they begin to soften.

2. Add the chicken thigh pieces to the skillet and cook for 5 to 7 minutes, or until the chicken is fully cooked. Stir often to ensure even cooking.

3. Add the garlic and ginger to the skillet and cook for about 1 minute, or until fragrant.

4. Stir in the coconut milk and Thai curry paste and season with salt and pepper.

5. Reduce the heat to medium and simmer the mixture for about 5 minutes to thicken it.

6. Stir in the spinach and lime juice and cook for 1 to 2 more minutes, just until the spinach is wilted.

7. Serve over the cauliflower rice and garnish with cilantro (if using).

TIP Find red curry paste in the international aisle of your grocery store. My favorite brand is Thai Kitchen.

TIP I like buying Native Forest Simple Coconut Milk or making my own (page 184). Be sure to shake the container vigorously before opening to combine the coconut and water.

PER SERVING
Calories: 1,071; Total Fat: 92g; Total Carbs: 19g; Fiber: 4g; Net Carbs: 15g; Protein: 40g
Macronutrients: Fat: 77%; Protein: 15%; Carbs: 8%

Za'atar Chicken "Couscous" Bowl

PREP TIME: 10 MINUTES, PLUS 10 MINUTES TO OVERNIGHT TO MARINATE |
COOK TIME: 45 MINUTES

Za'atar seasoning is a classic Middle Eastern spice that is perfect to sprinkle on basically everything. It has an earthy and savory flavor that pairs perfectly with lemon and garlic. Serve this chicken on top of a keto-friendly version of couscous, and you've got yourself a meal that is both satisfying and healthy!

SERVES 2

¼ cup avocado oil

Juice from 1 lemon

4 garlic cloves, minced

2 tablespoons za'atar
  spice, divided

4 skin-on chicken thighs

2 cups cauliflower rice

1 tablespoon extra-virgin
  olive oil

1 teaspoon toasted
  pine nuts

1 teaspoon
  pomegranate seeds

1 teaspoon chopped
  fresh parsley

Pink Himalayan salt

Freshly ground
  black pepper

1. In a small bowl, combine the avocado oil, lemon juice, garlic, and 1 tablespoon of za'atar spice.

2. Place the chicken thighs in a shallow dish and pour the za'atar mixture on top. Cover and marinate in the refrigerator for at least 10 minutes and up to overnight.

3. Preheat the oven to 400°F.

4. Transfer the marinated chicken thighs to a baking dish or ovenproof skillet (like a cast iron). Sprinkle the remaining 1 tablespoon of za'atar spice onto the top of the chicken thighs.

5. Roast for 40 to 45 minutes.

6. While the chicken in roasting, cover the bottom of a sauté pan or skillet with a very thin layer of water over medium heat. Salt the water and bring to a simmer.

7. Add the cauliflower rice to the skillet, spreading it out in an even layer. Bring the water back up to a simmer, then reduce the heat to low. Place a lid on the skillet and steam for 5 minutes.

8. Transfer the steamed cauliflower to a bowl and fluff with a fork. Mix in the olive oil, toasted pine nuts, pomegranate seeds, and parsley. Season with salt and pepper. Serve alongside the roasted chicken thighs. Garnish with a sprinkle more of the za'atar spice on top.

TIP Find za'atar seasoning in the international aisle of the grocery store or make your own by combining: 1 tablespoon of ground cumin, 1 tablespoon of dried thyme, 1 tablespoon of sumac, 1 tablespoon of toasted sesame seeds, 1 teaspoon of pink Himalayan salt, 1 teaspoon of black pepper. This will yield about ⅓ cup, so store any extra in a sealed container in your pantry for up to 3 months.

TIP Find premade cauliflower rice in the produce section or make your own: Buy a whole cauliflower head, chop it into florets, and place the cauliflower florets in a food processor. Pulse until the mixture resembles rice.

PER SERVING
Calories: 794; Total Fat: 67g; Total Carbs: 13g; Fiber: 5g; Net Carbs: 8g; Protein: 36g
Macronutrients: Fat: 76%; Protein: 18%; Carbs: 6%

Chicken Salad Wraps, Two Ways

PREP TIME: 5 MINUTES | **COOK TIME:** 5 MINUTES

There are so many great chicken salad varieties available today—so I decided to include my two favorite versions. The base for the chicken salad is the same for both recipes, so you just need to decide the seasonings you'd like to use. If you don't want to make the homemade mayonnaise, feel free to use a clean brand like Primal Kitchen instead.

SUPER-QUICK
SERVES 1

FOR THE CHICKEN SALAD BASE

2 tablespoons Homemade Mayonnaise (page 188)
2 teaspoons lemon juice
Pink Himalayan salt
Freshly ground black pepper
2 boneless, skinless chicken thighs, poached and diced into ½-inch cubes
2 Bibb lettuce leaves

1. In a medium bowl, whisk together the mayonnaise and lemon juice. Season with salt and pepper.

2. Stir in the spices from your preferred version (either curry and garlic powder or tarragon and garlic powder).

3. Add the chicken and the remaining ingredients from your preferred version.

4. Stir well to coat. Ideally, refrigerate the chicken salad for an hour or before serving, so the flavors can meld together.

5. Spoon the chicken salad into the Bibb lettuce leaves and wrap to secure.

FOR THE
CURRY VERSION

1 teaspoon curry powder

½ teaspoon garlic powder

¼ cup diced celery

1 tablespoon
  chopped pecans

1 tablespoon finely
  chopped cilantro

FOR THE
TARRAGON VERSION

1 tablespoon fresh chopped
  tarragon, or 1 teaspoon
  dried tarragon

½ teaspoon garlic powder

¼ cup diced celery

5 grapes, halved

1 tablespoon
  chopped pecans

TIP Yes, there are grapes in the tarragon version of this chicken salad. While grapes are not traditionally a keto-friendly fruit, we are only using 5 of them here. One grape has only 0.4 grams of carbs, meaning that 5 grapes have only 2 grams—totally fine for keto.

PER SERVING (CHICKEN SALAD BASE)
Calories: 534; Total Fat: 42g; Total Carbs: 1g; Fiber: 0g; Net Carbs: 1g; Protein: 33g
Macronutrients: Fat: 71%; Protein: 25%; Carbs: 4%

Sheet Pan Chicken and Broccolini

PREP TIME: 5 MINUTES | **COOK TIME:** 45 MINUTES

Who doesn't love a sheet pan meal? You just throw everything on a baking sheet and let the oven do all the work—no mess and no fuss. This recipe features chicken thighs and broccolini, which are a great combination together.

ELIMINATION-FRIENDLY

SERVES 1

2 tablespoons avocado
   oil, divided
1 tablespoon
   balsamic vinegar
1 tablespoon
   coconut aminos
Pink Himalayan salt
Freshly ground
   black pepper
2 skin-on chicken thighs
½ bunch broccolini (about
   6 stalks)
4 garlic cloves, minced

1. Preheat the oven to 400°F. Line a baking sheet with parchment paper.

2. In a medium bowl, whisk together 1 tablespoon of avocado oil, the balsamic vinegar, and coconut aminos. Season with salt and pepper. Add the chicken thighs to the bowl and use a spoon to fully coat all sides with the sauce.

3. Transfer the chicken thighs to your lined baking sheet, skin-side down. Roast for 30 minutes.

4. In a medium bowl, mix together the broccolini, garlic cloves, and the remaining 1 tablespoon of avocado oil. Season with salt and pepper. Toss to fully coat the broccolini.

5. After 30 minutes, carefully remove the baking sheet and use a pair of tongs to flip the chicken skin-side up.

6. Arrange the broccolini mixture around the chicken thighs and put the baking sheet back in the oven for 15 more minutes, until the chicken is fully cooked.

TIP Broccolini is also known as "baby broccoli" and is similar to broccoli but with smaller florets and longer stalks. You can also use broccoli florets in this recipe.

PER SERVING
Calories: 732; Total Fat: 57g; Total Carbs: 9g; Fiber: 0g; Net Carbs: 9g; Protein: 36g
Macronutrients: Fat: 70%; Protein: 20%; Carbs: 10%

Crispy Lemon–Rosemary Spatchcock Chicken

PREP TIME: 10 MINUTES | **COOK TIME:** 40 MINUTES

The term "spatchcock" in cooking basically means to split a chicken so that it is flattened. If you've never used this technique, I urge you to try it! (Your butcher can also spatchcock your chicken for you.) By flattening it, the chicken cooks faster and more evenly, plus you get the crispiest skin.

ELIMINATION-FRIENDLY

SERVES 4 TO 6

6 tablespoons ghee
4 tablespoons minced fresh
    rosemary
Zest from 2 lemons
8 garlic cloves, minced
1 (4-pound) whole chicken,
    spatchcocked
Pink Himalayan salt
Freshly ground
    black pepper
2 tablespoons lemon juice

1. Preheat the oven to 450°F.

2. In a medium bowl, combine the ghee, rosemary, lemon zest, and garlic cloves.

3. Place the chicken skin-side up on a rimmed baking sheet or in a cast iron skillet (if it fits). Pat the chicken dry with paper towels and season with salt and pepper.

4. Gently lift the skin of the chicken using your fingers and rub 4 tablespoons of the ghee mixture under the skin, spreading the rest of the mixture on top of the skin.

5. Roast the chicken for 10 minutes, then reduce the heat to 400°F and bake for another 30 to 40 minutes, or until a meat thermometer inserted in thickest portion of the chicken reads 165°F.

6. Drizzle the lemon juice over the chicken and let it rest for 10 minutes before slicing and serving.

TIP To spatchcock, place the bird on a cutting board with its backbone facing you. Remove the backbone by using a sharp pair of scissors to cut along both sides of the spine. Then pull out the backbone and press down on the breasts to flatten. Save the backbone in your freezer to make Healing Bone Broth (page 183).

PER SERVING (1 OF 4 TOTAL)
Calories: 1,063; Total Fat: 80g; Total Carbs: 9g; Fiber: 1g; Net Carbs: 8g; Protein: 86g
Macronutrients: Fat: 68%; Protein: 32%; Carbs: 3%

Butter Chicken

PREP TIME: 5 MINUTES | **COOK TIME:** 25 MINUTES

Butter chicken is a classic Indian dish. Tender pieces of chicken are smothered in a creamy and decadent sauce that features traditional Indian spices, coconut milk, and tomato. This dish is seriously delicious.

SUPER-QUICK
NUT- AND SEED-FREE
SERVES 1

3 tablespoons avocado
 oil, divided
2 boneless, skinless
 chicken thighs, cut into
 1-inch pieces
Pink Himalayan salt
Freshly ground
 black pepper
¼ yellow onion,
 finely chopped
2 garlic cloves, minced
½ tablespoon
 garam masala
½ teaspoon curry powder
½ teaspoon
 cayenne pepper
¼ teaspoon turmeric
½ cup full-fat unsweetened
 coconut milk
2 teaspoons tomato paste
1 cup cauliflower rice
1 teaspoon finely chopped
 fresh cilantro (optional)

1. In a medium sauté pan or skillet, heat 1 tablespoon of avocado oil over medium heat.

2. Add the chicken pieces, season with salt and pepper, and cook for 5 to 7 minutes, or until cooked through. Remove the chicken from the skillet and set aside.

3. Add 1 tablespoon of avocado oil to the same skillet.

4. Add the onion and garlic and cook for 3 to 5 minutes, or until softened and fragrant.

5. Add the garam masala, curry powder, cayenne, turmeric, coconut milk, and tomato paste, stir to combine, and simmer for 10 minutes.

6. Transfer the cooked chicken back to the skillet and stir to fully combine. Simmer for another 5 minutes.

7. In a separate skillet, heat the remaining 1 tablespoon of avocado oil. Add the cauliflower rice, season with salt, and cook for about 5 minutes, stirring frequently until the cauliflower softens.

8. Transfer the cauliflower to a bowl, top with the butter chicken, and garnish with chopped cilantro (if using).

TIP Garam masala can be found in the dried spice aisle of your local grocery store or you can purchase it online. It is made from a blend of ground spices used regularly in Indian cuisine.

TIP I like buying Native Forest Simple Coconut Milk or making my own (page 184). Be sure to shake the container vigorously before opening to combine the coconut and water.

TIP Find premade cauliflower rice in the produce section or make your own: Buy a whole cauliflower head, chop it into florets, and place the cauliflower florets in a food processor. Pulse until the mixture resembles rice.

PER SERVING
Calories: 932; **Total Fat:** 78g; **Total Carbs:** 18g; **Fiber:** 5g; **Net Carbs:** 13g; **Protein:** 38g
Macronutrients: Fat: 75%; Protein: 16%; Carbs: 9%

Sage-Roasted Turkey

PREP TIME: 5 MINUTES | **COOK TIME:** 20 MINUTES

It can be Thanksgiving any night of the week with this sage-roasted turkey. Turkey pairs perfectly with the citrusy, pine flavor of sage. I love serving this with my Horseradish Cauliflower Mash (page 99) and Thyme-Roasted Onions (page 104) for a nourishing, cozy dinner.

SUPER-QUICK
ELIMINATION-FRIENDLY
SERVES 1

1 tablespoon avocado oil
1 tablespoon chopped
   fresh sage
2 garlic cloves, minced
1 (6-ounce) turkey
   breast cutlet
Pink Himalayan salt
Freshly ground
   black pepper

1. Preheat the oven to 375°F. Line a baking sheet with parchment paper.

2. In a small bowl, combine the avocado oil, sage, and garlic.

3. Place the turkey on the lined baking sheet and season with salt and pepper. Fully coat the turkey with the sage mixture.

4. Bake for 15 to 20 minutes, or until fully cooked.

TIP Turkey cutlets are just pounded (or thinly sliced cuts of) turkey breast. If you can't find cutlets at your local grocery store, you can buy a turkey breast and pound it yourself: Wrap the turkey breast in plastic wrap, place it on a cutting board, and then use a meat tenderizer or the bottom of a heavy skillet to pound it until it is only about ¼-inch thick.

PER SERVING
Calories: 321; Total Fat: 15g; Total Carbs: 2g; Fiber: 0g; Net Carbs: 2g; Protein: 43g
Macronutrients: Fat: 42%; Protein: 54%; Carbs: 4%

Zucchini Turkey Burgers

PREP TIME: 5 MINUTES | **COOK TIME:** 10 MINUTES

Adding grated zucchini to your burger ensures that it will turn out extra juicy. It is also a great way to sneak extra fiber and nutrients into your diet. Even though standard burger buns are not an option in the keto world, you can still enjoy a handheld burger with the help of a few crisp Bibb lettuce leaves. Just wrap the whole thing in the lettuce leaves and enjoy.

SUPER-QUICK
ELIMINATION-FRIENDLY
SERVES 1

1 tablespoon avocado oil
6 ounces ground turkey
½ cup grated zucchini
1 scallion, thinly sliced
1 garlic clove, minced
Pink Himalayan salt
Freshly ground
  black pepper
½ avocado, sliced
4 Bibb lettuce leaves

1. In a sauté pan or skillet, heat the avocado oil over medium heat.

2. In a large bowl, add the ground turkey, zucchini, scallion, and garlic. Season with salt and pepper to taste and then use your hands to mix until the ingredients are well incorporated.

3. Form the turkey mixture into 2 patties.

4. Add the turkey patties to the skillet and cook them until they are nicely browned on each side and are no longer pink in the center, about 5 minutes on each side.

5. Top the patties with the sliced avocado and wrap each one in 2 lettuce leaves.

TIP Dress your burger as you like with mustard, mayo, aioli, tomato slices, sprouts, or no-sugar-added pickles.

PER SERVING
Calories: 550; Total Fat: 39g; Total Carbs: 15g; Fiber: 8g; Net Carbs: 7g; Protein: 37g
Macronutrients: Fat: 64%; Protein: 27%; Carbs: 9%

Italian Turkey Bolognese

PREP TIME: 5 MINUTES | **COOK TIME:** 25 MINUTES

This Italian turkey Bolognese is simple to prepare and full of flavor. Look for dark meat turkey; it has a higher fat content and doesn't dry out when you cook it. This recipe uses a combination of fresh and dried herbs to give it an Italian flair.

SUPER-QUICK
NUT- AND SEED-FREE
SERVES 1

½ zucchini, spiralized into ribbons or noodles
2 tablespoons avocado oil
¼ yellow onion, diced
2 garlic cloves, minced
6 ounces ground turkey
½ cup tomato sauce
2 teaspoons chopped basil, plus more for garnish
1 teaspoon dried oregano
¼ teaspoon red pepper flakes

1. Preheat the oven to 300°F. Line a baking sheet with parchment paper.

2. Place your zucchini in a single layer on the lined baking sheet and bake for 10 minutes to help evaporate any extra moisture.

3. In a large sauté pan or skillet, heat the avocado oil over medium-high heat. Add the onion and garlic and cook for 3 to 4 minutes, or until soft.

4. Add the ground turkey and cook until it's no longer pink, 5 to 7 minutes.

5. Add the tomato sauce, basil, oregano, and pepper flakes. Stir to combine.

6. Reduce the heat to low and simmer for 15 minutes.

7. Serve over the zucchini noodles and garnish with fresh basil.

TIP If you don't have a spiralizer, you can buy one online for $20 to $30. Alternatively, you can use a veggie peeler to peel the zucchini lengthwise into thin ribbons resembling noodles.

PER SERVING
Calories: 611; Total Fat: 43g; Total Carbs: 19g; Fiber: 4g; Net Carbs: 15g; Protein: 37g
Macronutrients: Fat: 63%; Protein: 24%; Carbs: 13%

Taco Zucchini Boats

PREP TIME: 5 MINUTES | **COOK TIME:** 20 MINUTES

Who needs a taco shell when you have zucchini? By hollowing out the center of a zucchini half, you have the perfect vessel to stuff with a delicious turkey taco mixture. You can eat this dish with a knife and fork, or if you want to fully commit—pick it up and eat it like a taco! Just make sure you have plenty of napkins on hand.

SUPER-QUICK
NUT- AND SEED-FREE
SERVES 2

1 zucchini
2 tablespoons avocado
  oil, divided
¼ yellow onion, diced
2 garlic cloves, minced
12 ounces ground turkey
1 teaspoon Mexi-Ranch
  Seasoning (page 181)
1 tablespoon tomato paste
¼ cup filtered water
½ avocado, diced
1 teaspoon chopped fresh
  cilantro

1. Preheat the oven to 400°F. Line a baking sheet with parchment paper.

2. Remove the ends from the zucchini and halve it lengthwise. Use a spoon to scoop out the seeds and center from both of the zucchini halves. Make sure to keep the sides intact.

3. Place the zucchini halves on the lined baking sheet and fully coat with 1 tablespoon avocado oil.

4. Roast the zucchini for 10 to 15 minutes, or until tender.

5. Meanwhile, in a medium sauté pan or skillet, heat the remaining 1 tablespoon of avocado oil over medium-high heat. Add the onion and garlic and cook for 3 to 4 minutes, or until soft.

6. Add the ground turkey and cook until it's no longer pink, 5 to 7 minutes.

7. Add the seasoning and stir to combine.

8. Add the tomato paste and water and bring to a gentle boil. Reduce the heat to low and simmer for 5 minutes.

9. Spoon the turkey mixture into the roasted zucchini and bake 5 minutes longer.

10. Remove from the oven and garnish with avocado and cilantro. For more of a kick, add hot sauce, diced onions, or sliced jalapeños.

PER SERVING
Calories: 479; **Total Fat:** 33g; **Total Carbs:** 12g; **Fiber:** 5g; **Net Carbs:** 7g; **Protein:** 36g
Macronutrients: Fat: 62%; Protein: 30%; Carbs: 8%

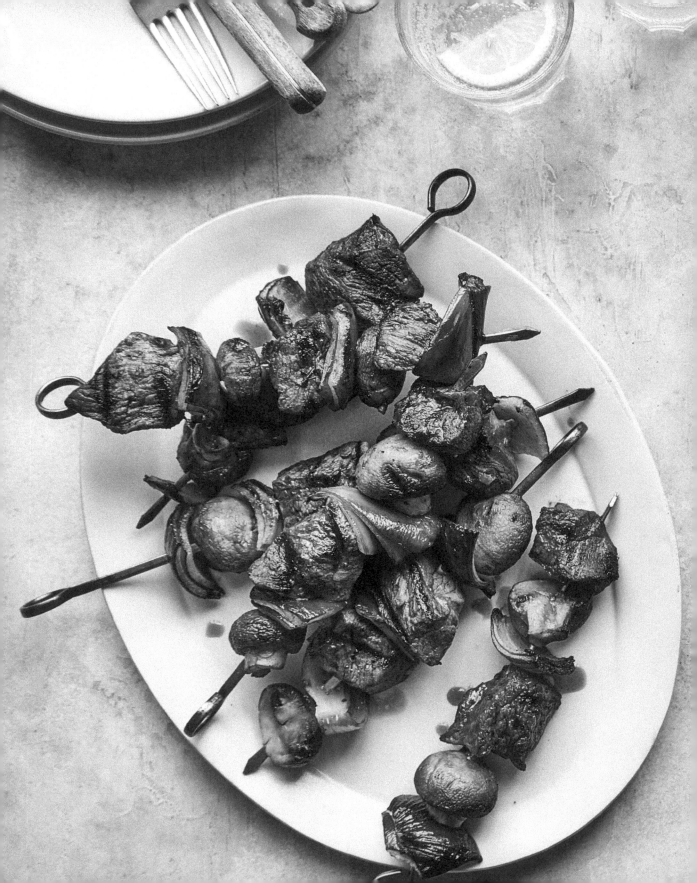

CHAPTER NINE

Beef, Pork, and Lamb

Chinese Beef Skewers

PREP TIME: 5 MINUTES, PLUS 3 HOURS TO MARINATE | COOK TIME: 10 MINUTES

When I was in elementary school, we would get Chinese food every Friday night. My favorite thing to order was the pupu platter, which was essentially a tray of appetizers. I absolutely loved the beef skewers. This recipe is my keto homage to a childhood favorite, and dare I say . . . it even tastes better than the original.

SUPER-QUICK
ELIMINATION-FRIENDLY
SERVES 1

1 tablespoon
balsamic vinegar

2 teaspoons
coconut aminos

1 teaspoon grated
ginger root

2 tablespoons avocado oil

1 garlic clove, minced

1 (6-ounce) beef sirloin, cut
into 1-inch pieces

¼ red onion, cut into
1-inch pieces

2 skewers (metal, or
wooden soaked in water
for 1 hour)

1. Mix the vinegar, coconut aminos, ginger, avocado oil, and garlic in a shallow baking dish.

2. Add the beef cubes and stir to fully coat.

3. Cover the dish with plastic wrap and refrigerate for at least 3 hours.

4. Preheat a grill pan over medium heat.

5. Thread 6 onion pieces and 6 beef cubes on each skewer, alternating between the two.

6. Grill the kebabs for 3 to 5 minutes on each side.

TIP If you don't have skewers, you can cook the sirloin cubes and onions in a skillet instead and serve them over some cauliflower rice.

PER SERVING
Calories: 638; Total Fat: 42g; Total Carbs: 8g; Fiber: 1g; Net Carbs: 7g; Protein: 52g
Macronutrients: Fat: 59%; Protein: 33%; Carbs: 8%

Steak Shish Kebabs

PREP TIME: 10 MINUTES, PLUS 10 MINUTES TO OVERNIGHT TO MARINATE | **COOK TIME:** 10 MINUTES

I love a good shish kebab. I mean what is better than a skewer full of meat and veggies? It is essentially a handheld meal. This recipe serves one, but it can be easily multiplied to serve as many people as you like.

SUPER-QUICK
NUT- AND SEED-FREE
SERVES 1

2 tablespoons avocado oil, divided, plus more for brushing the grill

1 tablespoon coconut aminos

1 teaspoon lemon juice

1 teaspoon red wine vinegar

1 teaspoon Dijon mustard

1 garlic clove, minced

1 (6-ounce) sirloin steak, cut into 1-inch pieces

4 white button mushrooms, halved (if small, keep them whole)

½ green bell pepper, cut into 1-inch pieces

¼ red onion, cut into 1-inch pieces

Pink Himalayan salt

Freshly ground black pepper

2 skewers (metal, or wooden soaked in water for 1 hour)

1. In a small bowl, combine 1 tablespoon of avocado oil, coconut aminos, lemon juice, red wine vinegar, Dijon mustard, and garlic.

2. Place the steak in a shallow dish and pour the marinade on top. Cover and marinate in the refrigerator for at least 10 minutes and up to overnight.

3. Preheat a grill pan over medium heat and brush it with avocado oil.

4. In a medium bowl, toss the mushrooms, peppers, and red onion in the remaining 1 tablespoon of avocado oil. Season with salt and pepper.

5. Thread the marinated steak and vegetables onto the skewers, alternating each one.

6. Grill the kebabs for 3 to 5 minutes on each side.

TIP Make sure you cut your ingredients into the same size so everything cooks uniformly. Also, leave some space between each ingredient on the skewer so they can cook in the middle.

PER SERVING
Calories: 670; Total Fat: 42g; Total Carbs: 13g; Fiber: 3g; Net Carbs: 10g; Protein: 55g
Macronutrients: Fat: 56%; Protein: 33%; Carbs: 11%

Deconstructed Burger Salad

PREP TIME: 5 MINUTES | COOK TIME: 10 MINUTES

This salad is basically just a burger served in a bowl and it tastes just as good, if not better than the original. This recipe includes all the classic burger toppings: mustard, pickles, tomatoes, and onions and is then finished off with a classic ranch dressing. This salad is guaranteed to become a family favorite.

SUPER-QUICK
NUT- AND SEED-FREE
SERVES 1

1 tablespoon avocado oil
6 ounces ground beef
1 garlic clove, minced
1 teaspoon yellow mustard
½ teaspoon dill pickle juice
2 cups romaine
  lettuce, chopped
4 cherry tomatoes, halved
1 tablespoon diced
  red onion
1 tablespoon diced dill
  pickle spears
¼ cup Classic Ranch
  Dressing (page 180)

1. In a sauté pan or skillet, heat the avocado oil over medium heat.
2. Add the ground beef and garlic to the skillet and cook for about 5 minutes, stirring often and breaking down the meat.
3. Stir in the mustard and pickle juice and cook for another minute.
4. In a bowl, add the romaine, tomatoes, red onion, and pickles. Pour in the dressing and toss well.

TIP When buying pickles for this recipe, check the food label to ensure that there are no added sugars on the ingredients list.

PER SERVING
Calories: 1,459; Total Fat: 139g; Total Carbs: 12g; Fiber: 3g; Net Carbs: 9g; Protein: 35g
Macronutrients: Fat: 86%; Protein: 10%; Carbs: 4%

Keto Chili

PREP TIME: 5 MINUTES | **COOK TIME:** 20 MINUTES, PLUS 1 TO 2 HOURS SIMMER TIME

If you are looking for a worthy crowd-pleaser on game day, you've come to the right place. Make sure you adjust the recipe for how many people you are feeding. This chili comes together in one large stockpot. You can easily make it in advance and keep it warm on the stovetop until you're ready to serve it.

SUPER-QUICK
NUT- AND SEED-FREE
SERVES 2

1 tablespoon avocado oil
½ yellow onion, diced
2 garlic cloves, minced
1 jalapeño pepper, chopped (less if you don't want it super spicy!)
6 ounces ground beef
6 ounces ground pork
2 teaspoons ground cumin
1 teaspoon chili powder
2 cups crushed tomatoes
1 avocado, diced (optional)
Fresh cilantro, for garnish (optional)
Scallions, thinly sliced, for garnish (optional)

1. In a medium stockpot, heat the avocado oil over medium-high heat. Add the onion, garlic, and jalapeño and cook for 3 to 4 minutes, or until soft.

2. Add the ground beef and ground pork and cook for about 5 minutes, stirring often and breaking down the meat.

3. After 5 minutes, add the cumin and chili powder and cook for another 2 to 3 minutes, or until the meat is fully cooked.

4. Stir in the tomatoes and bring to a boil. Then reduce the heat to low and simmer for 1 to 2 hours.

5. Garnish with the avocado, cilantro, and scallions (if using).

TIP This chili freezes really well. Let it cool and then transfer it to a sealed container with an airtight lid. Store it in the freezer for up to 2 months.

PER SERVING
Calories: 621; Total Fat: 48g; Total Carbs: 13g; Fiber: 3g; Net Carbs: 10g; Protein: 38g
Macronutrients: Fat: 70%; Protein: 24%; Carbs: 6%

Thai Beef Curry with Coconut Rice

PREP TIME: 10 MINUTES | **COOK TIME:** 30 MINUTES

I love the versatility of Thai curries. This Thai beef curry is perfect comfort food that has just enough spice to warm you up on a cold winter night. The spice of the curry pairs perfectly with the sweet coconut rice. This combination is out of this world.

NUT- AND SEED-FREE
SERVES 1

FOR THE CURRY

1 tablespoon coconut oil

½ cup red bell pepper, thinly sliced

¼ cup yellow onion, thinly sliced

1 (6-ounce) beef tenderloin, thinly sliced

½ cup full-fat, unsweetened coconut milk

2 teaspoons Thai red curry paste

1 teaspoon coconut aminos

1 teaspoon fish sauce

Pink Himalayan salt

Freshly ground black pepper

½ cup fresh Thai basil leaves or regular basil

1 tablespoon lime juice

1. In a medium sauté pan or skillet, heat the coconut oil over medium-high heat. Add the pepper and onion and sauté for 3 to 4 minutes, or until they begin to soften.

2. Add the beef slices to the skillet and cook for about 5 minutes, or until the beef is fully cooked. Stir often to ensure even cooking.

3. Stir in the coconut milk, Thai curry paste, coconut aminos, and fish sauce, and season with salt and pepper.

4. Reduce the heat to medium and simmer for about 5 minutes to thicken. Stir in the basil leaves and lime juice and keep warm on the stovetop while you make the coconut rice.

5. In another medium sauté pan or skillet, heat the coconut oil over medium-high heat. Add the shredded coconut and sauté for 1 minute, stirring continuously so it doesn't burn.

6. Add the cauliflower rice and sauté for 2 to 3 minutes.

7. Stir in half of the coconut cream and cook for 5 minutes then add the other half of the coconut cream. Season with salt.

FOR THE COCONUT RICE

1 tablespoon coconut oil
1 tablespoon unsweetened
 shredded coconut
1 cup cauliflower rice
¼ cup coconut cream
Pink Himalayan salt

8. Cook, stirring occasionally for another 5 to 10 minutes, or until the cauliflower is cooked through.

9. Transfer the cauliflower rice to a bowl and top with the beef curry.

TIP Find red curry paste in the international aisle of your grocery store. My favorite brand is Thai Kitchen.

TIP I like buying Native Forest Simple Coconut Milk or making my own (page 184). Be sure to shake the container vigorously before opening to combine the coconut and water.

TIP Find premade cauliflower rice in the produce section or make your own: Buy a whole cauliflower head, chop it into florets, and place the cauliflower florets in a food processor. Pulse until the mixture resembles rice.

PER SERVING
Calories: 942; Total Fat: 62g; Total Carbs: 35g; Fiber: 5g; Net Carbs: 30g; Protein: 61g
Macronutrients: Fat: 59%; Protein: 26%; Carbs: 15%

Ground Beef Burrito Bowls

PREP TIME: 5 MINUTES | **COOK TIME:** 15 MINUTES

I love burrito bowls. It's so much fun to mix and match the ingredients. The combination here is probably my favorite, but sometimes I swap out the ground beef for shredded chicken. I've also been known to substitute the mixed greens for Cilantro-Lime Cauliflower Rice (page 92). Be as creative as you like and discover your favorite burrito bowl combo.

SUPER-QUICK
NUT- AND SEED-FREE
SERVES 1

1 tablespoon avocado oil
¼ red onion, diced
6 ounces ground beef
1 tablespoon Mexi-Ranch
    Seasoning (page 181)
2 cups mixed greens
½ avocado, diced
4 cherry tomatoes, halved
1 teaspoon chopped fresh
    cilantro (optional)

1. In a sauté pan or skillet, heat the avocado oil over medium-high heat.

2. Add the onion and sauté 5 to 7 minutes, or until soft.

3. Add the ground beef and cook until it's no longer pink, breaking the meat into small pieces as it cooks, about 5 minutes.

4. Add the seasoning and stir the mixture constantly for about 1 minute.

5. In a bowl, place the mixed greens and add the beef mixture. Top with the avocado, tomatoes, and cilantro (if using).

TIP If you are making this recipe ahead of time, make the ground beef mixture and store it in a sealed container in the refrigerator. Don't assemble the salad or cut the avocados and tomatoes until you are ready to serve.

PER SERVING
Calories: 870; Total Fat: 74g; Total Carbs: 20g; Fiber: 12g; Net Carbs: 8g; Protein: 34g
Macronutrients: Fat: 77%; Protein: 16%; Carbs: 7%

Skirt Steak with Cilantro Sauce

PREP TIME: 10 MINUTES, PLUS 10 MINUTES TO OVERNIGHT TO MARINATE | COOK TIME: 20 MINUTES

Grilling might just be one of the best ways to cook a skirt steak. It is a great cut for marinating and it cooks quickly, resulting in a tender and juicy steak each time. I love serving this grilled steak with a fresh and vibrant cilantro sauce.

SUPER-QUICK
ELIMINATION-FRIENDLY
SERVES 1

FOR THE STEAK

2 teaspoons fresh lime juice

1 teaspoon chopped fresh cilantro

1 teaspoon grated ginger root

1 garlic clove, minced

½ teaspoon coconut aminos

1 (6-ounce) skirt steak

FOR THE CILANTRO SAUCE

¼ cup fresh cilantro, finely chopped

1 teaspoon red wine vinegar

1 garlic clove, minced

2 tablespoons lime juice

2 tablespoons extra-virgin olive oil

1. In a small bowl, combine the lime juice, cilantro, ginger, garlic, and coconut aminos.

2. Place the steak in a shallow dish and pour on the marinade. Cover and marinate in the refrigerator for at least 10 minutes and up to overnight.

3. Remove the steak from the marinade and pat dry with a paper towel.

4. Heat your grill or grill pan to high.

5. Grill the steak for 4 to 6 minutes on each side and then remove the steak from the grill. Let it rest for 10 minutes.

6. Make the cilantro sauce. In a food processor or blender, place the cilantro, red wine vinegar, garlic, and lime juice; process to combine.

7. Slowly pour in the olive oil and pulse until smooth.

8. Drizzle the cilantro sauce over top of the steak or serve alongside the steak as a dipping sauce.

TIP Because skirt steak can be a little tough, your best bet is to tenderize it before cooking. To do that, simply place the skirt steak on a cutting board, cover it with plastic wrap, and then pound the heck out of it using a meat tenderizer or the bottom of a heavy skillet. Let it sit at room temperature for 20 minutes before cooking.

PER SERVING
Calories: 644; Total Fat: 49g; Total Carbs: 4g; Fiber: 1g; Net Carbs: 3g; Protein: 45g
Macronutrients: Fat: 68%; Protein: 28%; Carbs: 4%

Sheet Pan Fajitas

PREP TIME: 10 MINUTES | **COOK TIME:** 15 MINUTES

Fajitas are just so darn tasty. The smell, the taste, and now the easy cleanup because we are roasting all the ingredients on one baking sheet. I love using a flavorful piece of skirt steak as the centerpiece of this dish. It cooks fast and absorbs all the spices beautifully.

SUPER-QUICK
NUT- AND SEED-FREE
SERVES 1

1 (6-ounce) flank steak
½ red pepper, thinly sliced
½ poblano pepper,
   thinly sliced
¼ red onion, thinly sliced
2 tablespoons avocado oil
1 garlic clove, minced
1 teaspoon Mexi-Ranch
   Seasoning (page 181)
Juice of 1 lime
1 avocado, diced (optional)
Fresh cilantro, chopped,
   for topping (optional)

1. Preheat the oven to 450°F.

2. Lay the flank steak in the middle of a baking sheet. Arrange the red pepper, poblano pepper, and red onion around it.

3. In a small bowl, combine the avocado oil, garlic, and seasoning. Pour the spice mixture over the steak and vegetables and toss with your hands to fully coat.

4. Sprinkle the lime juice over the top of the steak and veggies.

5. Bake for 12 minutes, or until the steak has reached your desired level of doneness: rare (2 to 3 minutes per side), medium-rare (3 to 4 minutes per side), or medium-well (5 to 7 minutes per side).

6. Transfer the steak to a cutting board and let it rest for 10 minutes. Cut the steak into slices against the grain. Top with avocado and cilantro (if using).

TIP The fajitas taste great alongside Cilantro–Lime Cauliflower Rice (page 92).

PER SERVING
Calories: 559; Total Fat: 39g; Total Carbs: 13g; Fiber: 3g; Net Carbs: 10g; Protein: 38g
Macronutrients: Fat: 63%; Protein: 27%; Carbs: 10%

Glazed Lamb Chops

To many people, the thought of making lamb chops can be a very intimidating proposition but in reality, they are one of the easiest and tastiest cut of meats to prepare. Just broil them in the oven for about 10 minutes and you are done.

SUPER-QUICK
ELIMINATION-FRIENDLY
SERVES 1

1 tablespoon avocado oil
1 garlic clove, minced
1 teaspoon chopped
  fresh thyme
1 teaspoon chopped fresh
  rosemary
3 small-rib lamb chops
Pink Himalayan salt
Freshly ground
  black pepper

1. In a small bowl, combine the avocado oil, garlic, thyme, and rosemary.

2. Season the lamb chops well with salt and pepper and then coat the lamp chops with the herb mixture.

3. Set the oven to broil.

4. Place the lamb chops in a single layer on a broiling pan.

5. Place the pan on the top rack of the oven and broil the chops for 5 minutes, or until a deep golden brown.

6. Remove the pan from the oven and use a pair of tongs to flip over the lamb chops.

7. Place the pan back into the oven and broil again for 5 minutes. Remove from the heat.

8. Cover and rest for 5 minutes before enjoying.

TIP Make sure you flip the chops only once. You want to leave the lamb alone so that a nice golden crust forms on each side of the chop.

PER SERVING
Calories: 346; Total Fat: 25g; Total Carbs: 4g; Fiber: 1g; Net Carbs: 3g; Protein: 25g
Macronutrients: Fat: 65%; Protein: 29%; Carbs: 6%

Greek Lamb Meatballs with Mint Sauce

PREP TIME: 5 MINUTES | **COOK TIME:** 25 MINUTES

This dish is full of wonderful Greek flavors: mint, oregano, olives, and—of course—lamb. The meatballs are flavorful and delicious, plus super easy to make. Served over zucchini noodles tossed in a bright Mint Sauce, this dish will have everyone begging for seconds.

SUPER-QUICK
ELIMINATION-FRIENDLY
SERVES 1

FOR THE
ZUCCHINI NOODLES

½ zucchini, spiralized
    into noodles

FOR THE MEATBALLS

6 ounces ground lamb
1 teaspoon finely chopped
    fresh parsley
½ teaspoon finely chopped
    fresh mint
1 garlic clove, minced
1 teaspoon dried oregano
1 tablespoon avocado oil

1. Preheat the oven to 300°F. Line a baking sheet with parchment paper.

2. Place your zucchini in a single layer on the lined baking sheet and bake for 10 minutes to help evaporate any extra moisture.

3. Transfer the zucchini to bowl and set aside. Raise the temperature to 350°F and re-line the baking sheet with a fresh piece of parchment paper.

4. Make the meatballs. In a large bowl, mix the ground lamb, parsley, mint, garlic, and oregano until well combined.

5. Form the meat mixture into 1½-inch balls.

6. In medium-sized sauté pan or skillet, heat the avocado oil on high heat.

7. Place the meatballs in the skillet and sear on all sides for 5 to 10 minutes.

8. Transfer the seared meatballs to the baking sheet and bake for about 5 minutes, or until the internal temperature reaches about 130°F.

FOR THE MINT SAUCE

1 cups fresh basil
½ cup fresh mint
¼ cup pitted
  Kalamata olives
1 garlic clove, minced
¼ teaspoon pink
  Himalayan salt
2 tablespoons extra-virgin
  olive oil

9. Make the mint sauce. In a food processor, put the basil, mint, olives, garlic, and salt. Process continuously until the ingredients start to break down, about 30 seconds. Slowly pour in the oil and blend until the oil is fully incorporated.

10. Remove the sauce from the food processor bowl and toss with the zucchini.

11. Place the cooked meatballs on top. Garnish with extra olives and parsley.

TIP I love a good sear on these meatballs, but for easier cooking, you can skip the searing process and just oven-bake the meatballs at 400°F for about 15 minutes.

PER SERVING
Calories: 982; Total Fat: 90g; Total Carbs: 13g; Fiber: 4g; Net Carbs: 9g; Protein: 32g
Macronutrients: Fat: 82%; Protein: 13%; Carbs: 5%

Pork Chops with Gremolata

PREP TIME: 10 MINUTES | **COOK TIME:** 20 MINUTES

There is nothing better than a tender, juicy, pan-seared pork chop with a nice golden crust on the outside. I love topping the pork chop with an easy gremolata, which is an herb condiment made of lemon zest, garlic, and parsley. To add a hint of sweetness and some extra healthy fats, I have added toasted coconut to my gremolata and it is perfection!

SUPER-QUICK
ELIMINATION-FRIENDLY
SERVES 1

2 tablespoons unsweetened
   shredded coconut
1 (6-ounce) boneless
   pork chop
Pink Himalayan salt
Freshly ground
   black pepper
1 tablespoon avocado
   oil, divided
2 tablespoons finely
   chopped fresh parsley
1 teaspoon finely grated
   lemon zest

1. In a small sauté pan or skillet, put in the shredded coconut and cook over medium heat. Stir the coconut continuously until the coconut begins to lightly brown, 3 to 4 minutes. Transfer to a bowl and set aside to cool.

2. Pat the pork chop dry with paper towels and season with salt and pepper on both sides.

3. In a large overproof skillet (like a cast iron), heat the avocado oil over medium heat. Add the pork chop and cook for 2 to 3 minutes on each side.

4. Remove the pork chop and cover loosely with foil. Let it rest for 5 minutes and finish the gremolata.

5. In the same bowl as the toasted coconut, add the parsley and lemon zest. Season with salt and use your hands to mix together the ingredients and break up any lemon zest clumps.

6. Sprinkle the mixture over the rested pork chop.

TIP Use a Microplane to finely grate the peel of a lemon to create lemon zest. Also, the trick to a great gremolata is to release the oils from the lemon zest, which happens when you use your fingers to mix it.

PER SERVING
Calories: 410; Total Fat: 28g; Total Carbs: 4g; Fiber: 2g; Net Carbs: 2g; Protein: 32g
Macronutrients: Fat: 61%; Protein: 31%; Carbs: 8%

Balsamic–Thyme Pork Tenderloin

PREP TIME: 5 MINUTES | **COOK TIME:** 25 MINUTES

This is a dish that people will think you spent a lot of time preparing . . . but it takes only 30 minutes. Cooking the pork hot and fast in the oven results in maximum juiciness, and the balsamic and thyme taste amazing together and give major flavor to the tenderloin.

SUPER-QUICK
ELIMINATION-FRIENDLY
SERVES 4 TO 6

2 tablespoons
  balsamic vinegar
2 tablespoons avocado oil
2 thyme sprigs,
  leaves stripped and
  finely chopped
1 (2-pound) pork tenderloin
Pink Himalayan salt
Freshly ground
  black pepper

1. Preheat the oven to 475°F. Line a baking sheet with parchment paper.
2. In a small bowl, whisk together the balsamic vinegar, avocado oil, and thyme.
3. Place the pork tenderloin on the lined baking sheet and season with salt and pepper. Fully coat the pork with the vinegar mixture on all sides.
4. Roast for 20 to 25 minutes.
5. Remove the pork from the oven, transfer to a cutting board, and cover loosely with foil. Let the tenderloin rest for 5 minutes before slicing.

TIP Don't overcook your pork. To keep it nice and juicy, aim for an internal temperature of 145°F to 160°F.

PER SERVING
Calories: 525; Total Fat: 26g; Total Carbs: 1g; Fiber: 0g; Net Carbs: 1g; Protein: 67g
Macronutrients: Fat: 45%; Protein: 51%; Carbs: 4%

Slow Cooker Carnitas

PREP TIME: 10 MINUTES | **COOK TIME:** 20 MINUTES

This dish is extremely easy to make, thanks to a slow cooker. Your entire house will smell amazing as this cooks low and slow. This pairs perfectly with Cilantro–Lime Cauliflower Rice (page 92) for a satisfying meal.

NUT- AND SEED-FREE
SERVES 4 TO 6

1 (4-pound) boneless, skinless pork shoulder
Pink Himalayan salt
Freshly ground black pepper
1 tablespoon dried oregano
2 teaspoons ground cumin
1 red onion, thinly sliced
1 jalapeño pepper, diced
4 garlic cloves, minced
Juice of 1 lime

1. Rinse and dry the pork shoulder and season all sides with salt and pepper.

2. In a small bowl, combine the oregano and cumin and rub the mixture all over the pork.

3. Place the pork in a slow cooker (fat cap up) and add the onion, jalapeño, and garlic. Pour the lime juice on top.

4. Cook on low for 6 to 8 hours.

5. Remove the pork from the slow cooker, let it cool slightly, and then shred it using two forks.

TIP Traditional carnitas is usually "crisped" before eating. To crisp, heat 1 tablespoon of avocado oil in a large sauté pan or skillet over high heat. Spread the carnitas in the skillet and drizzle over some of the cooking juices. Cook until the juice evaporates and the bottom of the pork is golden brown. Flip the pork and cook for 1 to 2 minutes more. Depending on how much meat you are working with, you may need to crisp in batches.

PER SERVING
Calories: 933; Total Fat: 70g; Total Carbs: 15g; Fiber: 1g; Net Carbs: 14g; Protein: 65g
Macronutrients: Fat: 68%; Protein: 28%; Carbs: 4%

Egg Roll in a Bowl

PREP TIME: 5 MINUTES | **COOK TIME:** 20 MINUTES

In the keto world, everyone has their version of "egg roll in a bowl," and this is mine. I have taken all the flavors of a classic egg roll and turned them into a quick-and-easy low-carb dish, without the added sugars and grain-filled wrapper. I mean, the best part of the egg roll is the filling, right?

SUPER-QUICK

SERVES 1

1 tablespoon sesame oil
¼ cup diced yellow onion
1 garlic clove, minced
1 teaspoon grated
 ginger root
6 ounces ground pork
Pink Himalayan salt
Freshly ground
 black pepper
1½ cups cabbage coleslaw
 mix or shredded cabbage
1 teaspoon coconut aminos
1 scallion, finely sliced

1. In a large sauté pan or skillet, heat the sesame oil over medium heat.

2. Add the onion, garlic, and ginger, and sauté for 2 to 3 minutes. Add the pork and season with salt and pepper.

3. Continue cooking for 10 minutes. Once the pork is just about done cooking, stir in the coleslaw mix and coconut aminos.

4. Cook for an additional 3 to 5 minutes, or until the slaw has softened slightly but is still crisp.

5. Transfer to a plate and sprinkle with scallions.

TIP If you are looking to add a little spice, I highly recommend drizzling some of my Chili-Infused Oil (page 187) over the dish.

TIP Feel free to swap the ground pork for ground chicken.

PER SERVING
Calories: 625; Total Fat: 50g; Total Carbs: 13g; Fiber: 4g; Net Carbs: 9g; Protein: 31g
Macronutrients: Fat: 72%; Protein: 20%; Carbs: 8%

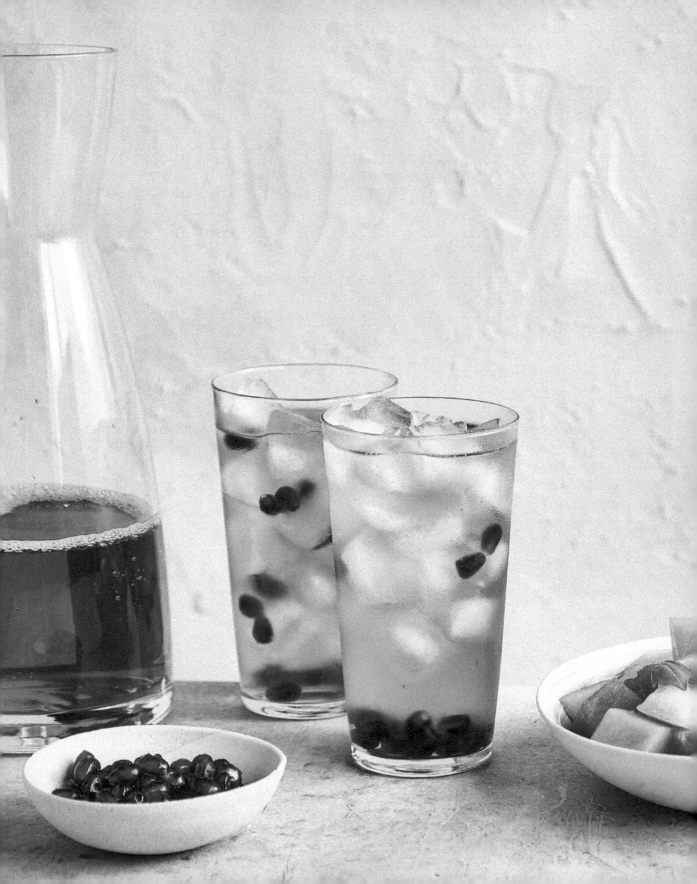

CHAPTER TEN

Beverages and Treats

ACV Spritz

PREP TIME: 10 MINUTES

Apple cider vinegar has many detoxifying and beneficial properties, including improving digestion, supporting the kidney and bladder, and aiding in weight loss. I love a good spritz, which I define as anything served with sparkling water in a wine glass over ice. So, say hello to my ACV spritz! Serve it in a wine glass for a cool, crisp, and classy feel.

SUPER-QUICK
ELIMINATION-FRIENDLY
VEGETARIAN
SERVES 1

¼ cup fresh mint leaves
1 cup sparkling water (such as Pellegrino)
1 tablespoon apple cider vinegar
Juice of ½ lemon
1 teaspoon grated ginger root
Ice cubes

1. Use the bottom of a spoon to muddle the mint leaves in the bottom of a wine glass.

2. Add the sparking water, apple cider vinegar, and lemon juice, and stir to combine.

3. Stir in the grated ginger.

4. Add your desired amount of ice.

TIP Swap out regular ice cubes for the Ginger-Turmeric Ice Cubes (page 186). They add more flavor and extra anti-inflammatory benefits.

PER SERVING
Calories: 34; Total Fat: 0g; Total Carbs: 5g; Fiber: 0g; Net Carbs: 0g; Protein: 0g
Macronutrients: Fat: 0%; Protein: 0%; Carbs: 100%

Cucumber and Lime Spa Water

PREP TIME: 10 MINUTES, PLUS 30 MINUTES COOLING TIME

Jazz up your water with fresh cucumber and lime slices. Cucumber is hydrating and can reduce bloating, and limes are great for digestion, making this water not only tasty but also great for you.

SUPER-QUICK
ELIMINATION-FRIENDLY
VEGETARIAN
SERVES 2

½ cucumber, sliced
1 lime, thinly sliced
6 cups cold filtered water
Ice cubes (optional)

1. Put the cucumber and lime in a pitcher. Then pour in the filtered water.

2. Transfer the pitcher to the refrigerator for 30 minutes to infuse the flavors.

3. Serve over ice (if using). Store in a covered container for 1 to 2 days in the refrigerator.

TIP Feel free to add any fresh herbs you have sitting around the refrigerator such as mint, basil, or cilantro.

PER SERVING
Calories: 20; Total Fat: 0g; Total Carbs: 6g; Fiber: 2g; Net Carbs: 4g; Protein: 1g
Macronutrients: Fat: 0%; Protein: 99%; Carbs: 1%

Iced Turmeric Tonic

PREP TIME: 10 MINUTES

I truly am in love with the anti-inflammatory benefits of turmeric, so I am always trying to figure out how to incorporate it into my diet. Black pepper also contains the bioactive compound piperine, which improves the body's ability to absorb curcumin (the anti-inflammatory powerhouse ingredient of turmeric). This iced tonic is refreshing and also a gorgeous orange color. Sweet cantaloupe adds subtle sweetness to this drink, while the ginger and turmeric add some zest.

SUPER-QUICK
ELIMINATION-FRIENDLY
VEGETARIAN
SERVES 1

½ cup cantaloupe, peeled, seeded, and cubed
1 (1-inch) piece ginger root, peeled and sliced
1 (1-inch) piece turmeric root, peeled and sliced, or 1 teaspoon turmeric powder
Freshly ground black pepper
1 cup filtered water
Ice cubes

1. Add the cantaloupe, ginger root, turmeric root, and a pinch of black pepper to a high-speed blender.
2. Blend until smooth. Add filtered water if needed.
3. Pour into a glass full of ice.

TIP A ½ cup of cubed raw cantaloupe has only 5.8 grams of net carbs, so stick to this serving size. Frozen cantaloupe works great in this recipe, too.

PER SERVING
Calories: 38; Total Fat: 1g; Total Carbs: 9g; Fiber: 1g; Net Carbs: 8g; Protein: 1g
Macronutrients: Fat: 24%; Protein: 11%; Carbs: 65%

Iced Pomegranate Green Tea

PREP TIME: 5 MINUTES, PLUS 1 TO 2 HOURS OF COOLING TIME | **COOK TIME:** 5 MINUTES

This is my favorite summer beverage. The earthy green tea pairs amazingly well with the sweet and tart pomegranate seeds. Pomegranates contain beneficial phytonutrients and antioxidants, plus they are very high in vitamin C, making them the perfect addition to this drink.

SUPER-QUICK
ELIMINATION-FRIENDLY
VEGETARIAN
SERVES 4

8 cups cold filtered water
4 green tea bags
1 cup pomegranate seeds
Ice cubes

1. In a saucepan, heat the filtered water until it comes to boil.
2. Add the green tea bags, turn off the heat, and steep for 5 minutes.
3. Pour the brewed tea into a pitcher and refrigerate for at least 1 to 2 hours or until cool.
4. Add the pomegranate seeds to the pitcher.
5. To serve, pour into a glass full of ice.

TIP Freeze your pomegranate seeds to make them extra refreshing. Pomegranate seeds have 6.4 grams of net carbs per ½ cup, so be sure to eat them in moderation.

PER SERVING
Calories: 36; Total Fat: 1g; Total Carbs: 8g; Fiber: 2g; Net Carbs: 6g; Protein: 1g
Macronutrients: Fat: 25%; Protein: 11%; Carbs: 64%

Chai Latte

PREP TIME: 5 MINUTES | **COOK TIME:** 15 MINUTES

This latte is rich and creamy and oh-so-satisfying. Traditional chai herbs like cardamom, cloves, peppercorns, cinnamon, and ginger give it a spicy kick. You can't beat fresh chai spices, but feel free to swap in an organic chai tea bag.

SUPER-QUICK
ELIMINATION-FRIENDLY
SERVES 1

5 cardamom pods
4 whole cloves
4 whole peppercorns
½ cup filtered water
1 cinnamon stick
1 (1-inch) piece ginger root, peeled and thinly sliced
1 cup full-fat unsweetened coconut milk
1 tablespoon collagen peptides
1 teaspoon MCT oil

1. Place the cardamom pods, cloves, and peppercorns in a resealable plastic bag and crush with a heavy sauté pan or skillet.
2. In a medium saucepan, heat the filtered water, crushed cardamom, crushed cloves, crushed peppercorns, cinnamon stick, and ginger root over medium-high heat and bring to a boil.
3. Reduce the heat to low and add the coconut milk.
4. Remove from the heat and steep the mixture for 10 minutes, then use a mesh strainer and carefully pour the strained chai tea mixture into a blender.
5. Add the collagen peptides and MCT oil.
6. Blend for 10 to 30 seconds, or until fully combined. Note: The liquids will be hot, so place a dish towel over the top of the blender lid before turning it on.
7. Pour the latte mixture into a large mug and serve.

TIP I like buying Native Forest Simple Coconut Milk or making my own (page 184). Be sure to shake the container vigorously before opening to combine the coconut and water.

TIP Collagen peptides are sourced from bovine hides or fish scales and are full of amino acids that help support the health of your body's connective tissue, skin, hair, and nails. They have no taste and come in powder form, making them great for smoothies or lattes. My favorite brand is Vital Proteins.

PER SERVING
Calories: 529; Total Fat: 48g; Total Carbs: 12g; Fiber: 2g; Net Carbs: 9g; Protein: 13g
Macronutrients: Fat: 82%; Protein: 10%; Carbs: 8%

London Fog Earl Grey Latte

PREP TIME: 5 MINUTES | COOK TIME: 5 MINUTES

This delicious "London Fog" latte (oddly created in Vancouver, Canada) is delicious and energizing. The bergamot oil in Earl Grey tea contains a powerful polyphenol that is known for its natural healing properties and for promoting cellular regeneration.

SUPER-QUICK
ELIMINATION-FRIENDLY
SERVES 1

½ cup filtered water
1 Earl Grey tea bag (make sure the only ingredients are black tea and bergamot oil)
1 tablespoon dried lavender (optional)
1 cup full-fat unsweetened coconut milk
1 teaspoon gluten-free vanilla extract
1 tablespoon collagen peptides
1 teaspoon MCT oil

1. Bring the water to a boil in a kettle or saucepan over high heat. Pour the boiling water into a large mug or teapot.

2. Add the tea bag and dried lavender (if using) to the water and steep for 4 to 5 minutes.

3. Meanwhile, heat the coconut milk and vanilla in a saucepan over medium heat until the mixture comes to a light simmer.

4. Once simmering, remove the saucepan from heat and transfer the coconut milk mixture to a blender. Add the collagen peptides and MCT oil.

5. Using a mesh strainer, pour the tea into the blender.

6. Blend for 10 to 30 seconds or until fully combined. Note: The liquids will be hot, so place a dish towel over the top of the blender lid before turning it on.

7. Pour the latte into a large mug and enjoy.

TIP Dried lavender adds aroma and flavor to any drink. You can buy it on Amazon or at stores such as World Market or a local herb shop. Make sure it's labeled for culinary use.

TIP See my tips on coconut milk and collagen peptides in the previous recipe.

PER SERVING
Calories: 514; Total Fat: 47g; Total Carbs: 7g; Fiber: 0g; Net Carbs: 7g; Protein: 12g
Macronutrients: Fat: 82%; Protein: 9%; Carbs: 9%

Coconut Matcha

This drink is packed with natural energy and healthy fats to keep you fueled. Matcha is also full of antioxidants, including epigallocatechin gallate (EGCG), which is thought to reduce inflammation, and is rich in fiber, chlorophyll, and other vitamins.

SUPER-QUICK
ELIMINATION-FRIENDLY
SERVES 1

1 teaspoon matcha powder
2 tablespoons hot filtered
    water (not boiling)
1 cup full-fat, unsweetened
    coconut milk
1 tablespoon collagen
    peptides
1 teaspoon MCT oil
Ground cinnamon,
    for garnish

1. In a small bowl, place the matcha powder. Add the water. Using the back of a spoon or a bamboo whisk, stir the mixture into a paste.

2. Meanwhile, heat the coconut milk in a saucepan over medium heat until it comes to a light simmer. Once simmering, remove the saucepan from heat and stir in the matcha paste.

3. Transfer the coconut-matcha mixture to a blender and add the collagen peptides and MCT oil.

4. Blend for 10 to 30 seconds or until fully combined. Note: The liquids will be hot, so place a dish towel over the top of the blender lid before turning it on.

5. Pour the matcha latte into a large mug and sprinkle with cinnamon. Enjoy immediately.

TIP For the coconut milk, I like buying Native Forest Simple Coconut Milk or making my own (page 184). Be sure to shake the container vigorously before opening to combine the coconut and water.

TIP Collagen peptides are sourced from bovine hides or fish scales and are full of amino acids that help support the health of your body's connective tissue, skin, hair, and nails. They have no taste and come in powder form, making them great for smoothies or lattes. My favorite brand is Vital Proteins.

PER SERVING
Calories: 508; Total Fat: 47g; Total Carbs: 6g; Fiber: 2g; Net Carbs: 4g; Protein: 14g
Macronutrients: Fat: 83%; Protein: 11%; Carbs: 6%

Signature Creamy Coffee

I intentionally excluded coffee from the keto cleanses because most people rely on it to wake up each day and I wanted to prove to you that you don't need it. But if you're someone who absolutely needs your coffee, feel free to swap this into some mornings of the cleanse. Coffee is actually an incredibly potent source of antioxidants and contains several important nutrients, such as riboflavin, manganese, potassium, and magnesium. My signature version of keto coffee is full of healthy fats that will keep you energized and satiated all morning.

SUPER-QUICK
VEGETARIAN
SERVES 1

1 cup brewed hot
   black coffee
1 cup full-fat, unsweetened
   coconut milk
½ tablespoon ghee
½ tablespoon MCT oil or
   coconut oil

1. Pour the coffee, coconut milk, ghee, and MCT oil or coconut milk into a blender.

2. Blend for 10 to 30 seconds or until fully combined and frothy. Note: The liquids will be hot, so place a dish towel over the top of the blender lid before turning it on.

3. Pour the latte mixture into a large mug and enjoy.

TIP Non-organic coffee crops are some of the most chemically treated plants in the world. It is crucial that you opt for organic versions whenever possible. And bonus points if you can find brands that test for the presence of mycotoxins (mold growing on the beans).

TIP For the coconut milk, I like buying Native Forest Simple Coconut Milk or making my own (page 184). Be sure to shake the container vigorously before opening to combine the coconut and water.

PER SERVING
Calories: 556; Total Fat: 56g; Total Carbs: 6g; Fiber: 0g; Net Carbs: 6g; Protein: 3g
Macronutrients: Fat: 91%; Protein: 2%; Carbs: 7%

Golden Milk

PREP TIME: 5 MINUTES | **COOK TIME:** 5 MINUTES

This healing golden milk is especially comforting on a cold winter's day. The turmeric, ginger, and cinnamon are a classic combination and provide a warming flavor. Black pepper also contains the bioactive compound piperine, which improves the body's ability to absorb curcumin (the anti-inflammatory powerhouse ingredient of turmeric). The coconut milk and the coconut oil provide plenty of medium-chain fatty acids that are easily absorbed and used by the body for fuel.

SUPER-QUICK
ELIMINATION-FRIENDLY
VEGETARIAN
SERVES 1

1½ cups full-fat, unsweetened coconut milk
2 teaspoons coconut oil
1 teaspoon ground turmeric
⅛ teaspoon ground ginger
⅛ teaspoon ground cinnamon
Freshly ground black pepper

1. In a saucepan, combine the coconut milk, coconut oil, turmeric, ginger, cinnamon, and a pinch pepper over medium heat and whisk to combine.
2. Remove from the heat when the liquid is hot, but not boiling.
3. Pour into a large mug and enjoy.

TIP For the coconut milk, I like buying Native Forest Simple Coconut Milk or making my own (page 184). Be sure to shake the container vigorously before opening to combine the coconut and water.

PER SERVING
Calories: 723; Total Fat: 73g; Total Carbs: 11g; Fiber: 1g; Net Carbs: 10g; Protein: 5g
Macronutrients: Fat: 91%; Protein: 3%; Carbs: 6%

Vanilla–Cinnamon Fat Bombs

PREP TIME: 20 MINUTES | **COOK TIME:** 5 MINUTES

These fat bombs are loaded with healthy fats and classic flavors like coconut, vanilla, and cinnamon, making for a satisfying afternoon snack.

SUPER-QUICK
MAKES 10 TO 12 FAT BOMBS

3 tablespoons coconut butter (also known as manna)

2 tablespoons ghee

2 tablespoons MCT oil

2 teaspoons gluten-free vanilla extract

⅔ cup almond flour

2 tablespoons collagen peptides

2 tablespoons coconut flour

2 teaspoons cinnamon

1 teaspoon pink Himalayan salt

1. In a saucepan, melt the coconut butter and ghee. Then combine the coconut butter, ghee, MCT oil, and vanilla extract over low heat then whisk to fully combine. Remove from the heat.

2. In a separate bowl, mix together the almond flour, collagen peptides, coconut flour, cinnamon, and salt.

3. Slowly pour the melted coconut butter mixture into the dry ingredients, stirring to remove any clumps.

4. Place the bowl in the freezer for 15 to 20 minutes, or until the dough resembles cookie dough.

5. Using a spoon, scoop out 1 tablespoon of the hardened dough, roll it into a ball with your hands, and transfer to a dinner plate in a single layer. Repeat.

6. Place the fat bombs on the plate in the freezer for 5 more minutes to fully set.

7. Transfer to a sealed container and store in the freezer for up to 7 days.

TIP I use Fourth & Heart's Madagascar Vanilla Bean ghee for this recipe to add a bit of sweetness.

TIP Collagen peptides are sourced from bovine hides or fish scales and are full of amino acids that help support the health of your body's connective tissue, skin, hair, and nails. They have no taste and come in powder form, making them great for smoothies or lattes. My favorite brand is Vital Proteins.

PER SERVING (2 FAT BOMBS)
Calories: 282; Total Fat: 24g; Total Carbs: 8g; Fiber: 5g; Net Carbs: 3g; Protein: 8g
Macronutrients: Fat: 76%; Protein: 11%; Carbs: 13%

Coconut–Lime Macaroons

PREP TIME: 5 MINUTES | **COOK TIME:** 12 MINUTES

Coconut and lime are a classic pairing. These macaroons take those flavors and combine them into an indulgent Elimination phase–compliant cookie that has amazing flavor and texture. No one will know that they are low-carb and anti-inflammatory.

SUPER-QUICK
ELIMINATION-FRIENDLY
MAKES 10 TO
12 MACAROONS

1 cup unsweetened
   shredded coconut
1 cup coconut butter
2 tablespoons collagen
   peptides
2 tablespoons coconut flour
1 tablespoon lime juice
1½ teaspoons lime zest,
   plus extra for garnish

1. Preheat the oven to 350°F. Line a baking sheet with parchment paper.

2. In a medium bowl, mix the coconut, coconut butter, collagen peptides, coconut flour, lime juice, and lime zest, using your hands to break apart any coconut butter clumps.

3. Roll the mixture into 1½-inch balls and place them on the baking sheet.

4. Bake the cookies for 10 to 12 minutes, or until the outsides start to brown.

5. Remove macaroons from the oven and garnish each with extra lime zest.

TIP If your dough is crumbly, add more coconut butter 1 teaspoon at a time until the dough stays compact.

TIP Collagen peptides are sourced from bovine hides or fish scales and are full of amino acids that help support the health of your body's connective tissue, skin, hair, and nails. They have no taste and come in powder form, making them great for smoothies or lattes. My favorite brand is Vital Proteins.

PER SERVING (2 MACAROONS)
Calories: 348; Total Fat: 31g; Total Carbs: 13g; Fiber: 8g; Net Carbs: 5g; Protein: 7g
Macronutrients: Fat: 80%; Protein: 8%; Carbs: 12%

Melon with Fresh Basil

PREP TIME: 10 MINUTES

Sweet melon paired with vibrant basil is a fabulous and refreshing appetizer or snack. Melon is a relatively low-carb fruit coming in at around 5 to 7 grams net carbs per ½ cup. It is also full of fiber, vitamin A, vitamin C, and beta-carotene, which is another reason why I love this dish.

SUPER-QUICK
ELIMINATION-FRIENDLY
VEGETARIAN
SERVES 4

2 cups cantaloupe, honeydew, or watermelon (or a combination)
1 cup basil leaves, torn
1 teaspoon fresh lime juice
½ teaspoon pink Himalayan salt

1. Cut the melon into 1-inch cubes and place in a medium bowl.
2. Top with the basil and lime juice and gently stir to combine.
3. Sprinkle with salt.
4. Scoop ½-cup portions into small bowls and enjoy immediately or shortly after preparing.

TIP For a fun presentation, use a melon baller or small cookie scoop to form perfectly shaped balls. The trick is to press the melon baller down into the melon until the fruit fills the entire scoop and then twist the melon ball right out.

PER SERVING (½ CUP)
Calories: 31; Total Fat: 0g; Total Carbs: 7g; Fiber: 1g; Net Carbs: 6g; Protein: 1g
Macronutrients: Fat: 0%; Protein: 13%; Carbs: 83%

Blackberries with Coconut Cream

PREP TIME: 10 MINUTES, PLUS OVERNIGHT COOLING TIME AND 30 MINUTES CHILL TIME

Blackberries are the perfect keto-friendly way to satisfy your sweet tooth. Top these blackberries with coconut whipped cream for the perfect dessert. For best results, chill the bowl and electric mixer beaters in the freezer for at least an hour before making the coconut whipped cream.

SUPER-QUICK
ELIMINATION-FRIENDLY
VEGETARIAN
SERVES 4

1 cup coconut cream, refrigerated overnight

2 teaspoons gluten-free vanilla extract

3 cups blackberries

1. In a medium bowl, use an electric mixer and beat the coconut cream and vanilla for 5 to 10 minutes, or until fluffy.

2. Refrigerate the whipped coconut cream for 30 minutes to firm it up more.

3. Top the blackberries with the chilled whipped cream.

TIP If you don't have coconut cream available, simply skim the solid white cream that rises to the top of a can of coconut milk when it is refrigerated.

PER SERVING (¾ CUP)
Calories: 182; Total Fat: 13g; Total Carbs: 14g; Fiber: 6g; Net Carbs: 8g; Protein: 1g
Macronutrients: Fat: 64%; Protein: 2%; Carbs: 34%

Strawberry Gummies

PREP TIME: 5 MINUTES, PLUS 6 HOURS COOLING TIME | COOK TIME: 5 MINUTES

These strawberry gummies are a delicious way to sneak beef gelatin into your diet. Gelatin can help ease joint pain, aid in digestive function, and improve skin health. Feel free to swap out blackberries or raspberries in this recipe to change up the flavor.

ELIMINATION-FRIENDLY

MAKES 20 GUMMIES

1 cup strawberries

⅓ cup water

1 tablespoon lemon juice

4 teaspoons beef gelatin powder

1. In a blender, purée the strawberries, water, and lemon juice until smooth.

2. Transfer the mixture to a small saucepan over medium-low heat and bring to a simmer.

3. Slowly whisk in the beef gelatin powder, making sure to break apart any clumps.

4. Continue heating the mixture until all of the ingredients are well combined and the gelatin is completely dissolved, 3 to 5 minutes.

5. Over a medium bowl, pour the mixture through a mesh strainer.

6. Place a silicone mold on a baking sheet and carefully pour the mixture into the mold.

7. Transfer the baking sheet to the refrigerator for at least 6 hours.

8. Pop the gummies out of the mold and store in a sealed container in the refrigerator for 1 to 2 weeks.

TIP Beef gelatin comes in powder form and is rich in collagen and amino acids, which are healing to your gut lining. When added to recipes, it acts as a thickener.

TIP You can find silicone molds on Amazon. If you don't have a silicone mold, you can use an ice cube tray instead.

PER SERVING (5 GUMMIES)
Calories: 23; Total Fat: 0g; Total Carbs: 3g; Fiber: 1g; Net Carbs: 2g; Protein: 3g
Macronutrients: Fat: 0%; Protein: 52%; Carbs: 48%

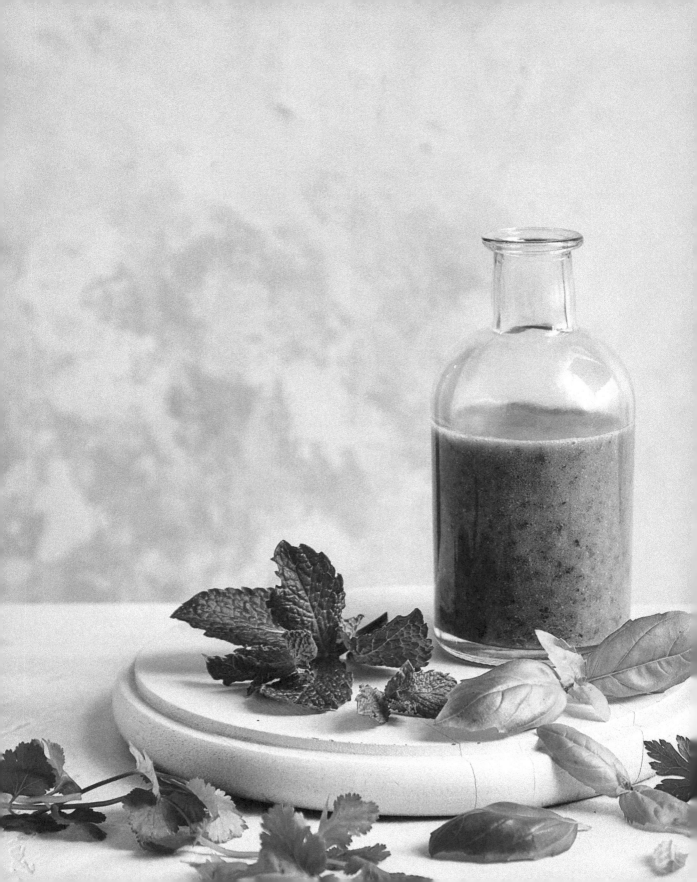

CHAPTER ELEVEN

Staples

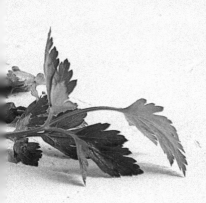

Dijon Vinaigrette

PREP TIME: 10 MINUTES

This dressing is one of my favorites. The tanginess of the red wine vinegar combined with the richness of the Dijon mustard make a wonderful combination. I added garlic to this recipe because I absolutely love it but feel free to leave it out—the dressing tastes great either way.

SUPER-QUICK
ELIMINATION-FRIENDLY
VEGETARIAN
MAKES ½ CUP

2 tablespoons red
   wine vinegar
1 tablespoon Dijon mustard
1 garlic clove, finely minced
¼ cup extra-virgin olive oil
Pink Himalayan salt
Freshly ground
   black pepper

1. In a small bowl, whisk the red wine vinegar, Dijon mustard, and garlic together until well combined.
2. Slowly drizzle in the olive oil and whisk until it emulsifies and thickens.
3. Season with salt and pepper to taste.
4. Store any leftover dressing in a sealed container in the refrigerator for up to 7 days. Shake the jar vigorously before using.

PER SERVING (¼ CUP)
Calories: 248; Total Fat: 27g; Total Carbs: 1g; Fiber: 0g; Net Carbs: 1g; Protein: 0g
Macronutrients: Fat: 98%; Protein: 0%; Carbs: 2%

Lemon Caesar Dressing

PREP TIME: 10 MINUTES | COOK TIME: 5 MINUTES

Caesar dressing is the absolute best. It's salty, tangy, creamy, and features classic flavors. The secret to a good Caesar dressing is anchovies. Don't be scared of anchovies; they are essential for the flavor of this dressing. You won't be able to taste them at all and (bonus!) anchovies are full of healthy fats and an excellent source of calcium, iron, and zinc.

SUPER-QUICK
ELIMINATION-FRIENDLY
MAKES 1 CUP

4 to 6 anchovy
   fillets, drained
2 garlic cloves
1 tablespoon Dijon mustard
2 egg yolks, room
   temperature
Zest of 2 lemons, room
   temperature
Juice of 2 lemons, room
   temperature
⅔ cup avocado oil

1. In a blender or food processor, put the anchovies, garlic, Dijon mustard, egg yolks, lemon zest, and lemon juice.

2. Process for 30 seconds or so, until smooth.

3. With the processor running, slowly pour the avocado oil into the food processor until the mixture emulsifies.

4. Store any leftover dressing in a sealed container in the refrigerator for up to 7 days.

TIP You can find anchovies in the grocery store in the same aisle you find canned tuna. Opt for anchovy fillets packed in olive oil.

PER SERVING (¼ CUP)
Calories: 388; Total Fat: 39g; Total Carbs: 3g; Fiber: 0g; Net Carbs: 3g; Protein: 2g
Macronutrients: Fat: 90%; Protein: 2%; Carbs: 8%

Ranch Dressing, Two Ways

PREP TIME: 10 MINUTES

Keto ranch dressing can easily be made at home in just a few minutes and tastes just as good as, if not better than, store-bought ranch dressings, which have added sugars and refined oils. This versatile recipe gives you two options: Classic or Mexi-ranch. Both can be used as a salad dressing or dip and they will soon become staples in your refrigerator.

CLASSIC RANCH

**SUPER-QUICK
ELIMINATION-FRIENDLY
VEGETARIAN**

MAKES 2 CUPS

MEXI-RANCH

**SUPER-QUICK
NUT- AND SEED-FREE
VEGETARIAN**

MAKES 2 CUPS

FOR THE RANCH DRESSING BASE

2 eggs, room temperature
¼ cup red wine vinegar
2 tablespoons seasoning
  blend of choice
1⅓ cups avocado oil
¼ cup full-fat,
  unsweetened
  coconut milk

1. In a blender or food processor, put the eggs, red wine vinegar, and seasoning.
2. Pulse a few times to combine the ingredients.
3. Start the blender or food processor and slowly pour in the avocado oil through the top.
4. Once all the oil has been incorporated, add the coconut milk and blend or pulse for a few more seconds.
5. Store any leftover dressing in a sealed container in the refrigerator for up to 7 days and store any leftover seasoning blend in a sealed container at room temperature for up to 6 months.

FOR THE CLASSIC RANCH SEASONING BLEND (YIELDS 10 TABLESPOONS)

6 tablespoons dried dill
1 tablespoon pink
 Himalayan salt
1 tablespoon freshly ground
 black pepper
1 tablespoon onion powder
1 tablespoon garlic powder

FOR THE MEXI-RANCH SEASONING BLEND (YIELDS 8 TABLESPOONS)

4 tablespoons cumin
1 tablespoon garlic powder
1 tablespoon chili powder
1 tablespoon onion powder
2 teaspoons dried oregano
2 teaspoons
 smoked paprika

TIP For the coconut milk, I like buying Native Forest Simple Coconut Milk or making my own (page 184). Be sure to shake the container vigorously before opening to combine the coconut and water.

PER SERVING (¼ CUP)
Calories: 758; Total Fat: 79g; Total Carbs: 3g; Fiber: 0g; Net Carbs: 3g; Protein: 4g
Macronutrients: Fat: 94%; Protein: 2%; Carbs: 4%

Green Goddess Dressing

This creamy, herb-filled dressing is not only amazing on salads but can also be used as a delicious dip. The fresh herbs give this dressing incredible depth of flavor as well as beautiful green color—hence the name. Feel free to mix and match the herbs based on what you have on hand.

SUPER-QUICK
ELIMINATION-FRIENDLY
VEGETARIAN
MAKES 2 CUPS

1 egg, room temperature
2 tablespoons lemon juice
⅔ cup avocado oil
2 tablespoons unsweetened
full-fat coconut milk
¼ cup basil leaves
¼ cup mint leaves
¼ cup parsley leaves
¼ cup cilantro leaves

1. In a blender or food processor, add the egg and lemon juice.

2. Pulse a few times to combine the ingredients.

3. Start the blender or food processor and slowly pour in the avocado oil through the top.

4. Once all the oil has been incorporated, add the coconut milk, basil, mint, parsley, and cilantro and blend or pulse for a few more seconds.

5. Store any leftover dressing in a sealed container in the refrigerator for up to 7 days.

TIP For the coconut milk, I like buying Native Forest Simple Coconut Milk or making my own (page 184). Be sure to shake the container vigorously before opening to combine the coconut and water.

PER SERVING (¼ CUP)
Calories: 188; Total Fat: 20g; Total Carbs: 1g; Fiber: 0g; Net Carbs: 1g; Protein: 1g
Macronutrients: Fat: 96%; Protein: 2%; Carbs: 2%

Healing Bone Broth

PREP TIME: 5 MINUTES | **COOK TIME:** 10 TO 24 HOURS

Bone broth is a staple in my kitchen. I make a big batch and keep it in the freezer to use in soups or to simply sip from a mug. It is gut-healing, nourishing, and has a rich, incredible depth of flavor. Make this recipe from just beef bones, just chicken bones, or a combination of both.

ELIMINATION-FRIENDLY

MAKES 20 CUPS

2 to 3 pounds raw beef
  bones, raw chicken
  bones, or a mix
1⅓ cups roughly
  chopped onion
1⅓ cups roughly
  chopped celery
1⅓ cups roughly
  chopped carrots
1 tablespoon apple
  cider vinegar
2 bay leaves
1 teaspoon pink
  Himalayan salt

1. Preheat the oven to 350°F.

2. In a large roasting pan, roast the bones for 30 minutes.

3. Transfer the bones to a large stockpot. Add the onion, celery, carrots, apple cider vinegar, bay leaves, and salt.

4. Fill the stockpot with enough filtered water so that the bones are covered by about 1 inch.

5. Bring the broth to a boil, then reduce to a simmer and cover.

6. After 2 hours, use a slotted spoon to skim off any impurities that float to the surface and discard them.

7. Cook the broth over the lowest heat for 8 to 24 hours.

8. Remove the broth from the heat and let it cool for 20 minutes or so.

9. Use a strainer to carefully remove the bones and vegetables.

10. Store your broth in a sealed container in the refrigerator for up to 5 days or freeze it for future use.

TIP Look for high-quality bones from grass-fed cattle and pastured chickens. To make a broth with the most collagen, try to use feet, knuckles, necks, and backs.

PER SERVING (1½ CUP)
Calories: 69; Total Fat: 4g; Total Carbs: 1g; Fiber: 0g; Net Carbs: 1g; Protein: 6g
Macronutrients: Fat: 52%; Protein: 35%; Carbs: 13%

Fresh Coconut Milk, Three Ways

I am obsessed with coconut milk! Although the full-fat canned version works great, it doesn't even come close to homemade coconut milk: There is just something about the taste and creaminess of it when it's freshly made. There are actually three different ways to make coconut milk. In each version, the fat (aka oils) in the coconut milk will separate from the water while it is in the refrigerator because there are no preservatives or fillers. Just shake or stir the coconut milk to combine before using. You may need to warm it up slightly to do this.

ELIMINATION-FRIENDLY
VEGETARIAN
MAKES 4 CUPS

METHOD 1

4 cups filtered water
2 cups unsweetened
    shredded coconut

METHOD 2

1 whole mature
    brown coconut
2 cups filtered water

METHOD 3

2 cups frozen fresh coconut
    meat (found in Asian
    supermarkets)
2 cups filtered water

METHOD 1   **PREP TIME:** 2 HOURS

1. In a saucepan, heat the filtered water over medium heat. When the water starts to simmer, remove it from the heat. You don't want to use boiling water.

2. Transfer the water to a large bowl and add the shredded coconut. Infuse for 1 to 2 hours.

3. Pour the coconut mixture into a high-speed blender. Blend on the highest speed for about 1 minute, or until the mixture is fully combined.

4. Over a large bowl, strain the coconut mixture through a nut milk bag or cheesecloth and squeeze out all the liquid.

5. Pour the liquid into a sealed container and store in the refrigerator for up to 3 days.

METHOD 2   **PREP TIME:** 15 MINUTES

1. Over a large bowl, carefully strike the coconut in a rhythmic motion, working your way around the whole coconut. Keep striking it until the shell cracks. The coconut water will start to drain out as you do this.

2. Once the coconut cracks open, use a paring knife to gently pry out the white coconut meat from the shell. Cut the coconut meat into 1-inch pieces.

3. Transfer the coconut meat pieces and the coconut water to a high-speed blender. Pour in the filtered water.

4. Blend on the highest speed for about 1 minute, or until the mixture is fully combined. It will be thick and not very smooth.

5. Over a large bowl, strain the coconut mixture through a nut milk bag or cheesecloth and squeeze out all the liquid.

6. Pour the liquid in a sealed container and store in the refrigerator for up to 3 days.

METHOD 3   **PREP TIME:** 8–10 HOURS

1. Thaw the frozen coconut meat in the refrigerator overnight.

2. Transfer the coconut meat and the filtered water to a high-speed blender.

3. Blend on the highest speed for about 1 minute, or until the mixture is fully combined. It will be thick and not very smooth.

4. Over a large bowl, strain the coconut mixture through a nut milk bag or cheesecloth and squeeze out all the liquid.

5. Pour the liquid in a sealed container and store in the refrigerator for up to 3 days.

PER SERVING, FLAKES (1 CUP)
Calories: 267; Total Fat: 27g; Total Carbs: 11g; Fiber: 5g; Net Carbs: 6g; Protein: 3g
Macronutrients: Fat: 91%; Protein: 4%; Carbs: 5%

PER SERVING, MEDIUM COCONUT OR 2 CUPS FROZEN (1 CUP)
Calories: 351; Total Fat: 33g; Total Carbs: 15g; Fiber: 9g; Net Carbs: 6g; Protein: 3g
Macronutrients: Fat: 85%; Protein: 3%; Carbs: 12%

Herb- and Fruit-Infused Ice Cubes

PREP TIME: 5 MINUTES, PLUS 5 HOURS FREEZE TIME

These infused ice cubes will add a burst of flavor to any drink and they are a great way use up extra herbs and produce before they go bad in your refrigerator. I love adding these ice cubes sparkling water, tea, and even smoothies.

ELIMINATION-FRIENDLY
VEGETARIAN
MAKES 12 ICE CUBES

FOR CUCUMBER-MINT

1 cup filtered water
1 cucumber, peeled
    and seeded
¼ cup fresh mint leaves
Pinch pink Himalayan salt

FOR STRAWBERRY-BASIL

1 cup filtered water
1 cup
    strawberries, trimmed
¼ cup fresh basil leaves
Pinch pink Himalayan salt

FOR GINGER-TURMERIC

1 cup filtered water
1 tablespoon fresh turmeric
    root, peeled and chopped
1 tablespoon peeled and
    chopped fresh ginger root

1. For each combination, put all the ingredients in a high-speed blender.

2. Blend on the highest speed for about 1 minute, or until the mixture is fully combined.

3. Transfer to an ice cube tray and freeze for at least 5 hours before using.

TIP You can also make these without the blender: Chiffonade your herbs and thinly slice your fruit. Fill your ice cube tray halfway with filtered water. Add the herbs and fruit to the tray compartments and use your fingers or a spoon to push them under the water. Put the half-filled ice cube tray into the freezer for 1 hour to set. Next, add some more water to the top of the cubes to fill the compartment up and freeze for 4 more hours.

PER SERVING, CUCUMBER-MINT (4 ICE CUBES)
Calories: 7; Total Fat: <1g; Total Carbs: 1g; Fiber: 1g; Net Carbs: 0g; Protein: <1g
Macronutrients: Fat: 0%; Protein: 0%; Carbs: 0%

PER SERVING, STRAWBERRY-BASIL (4 ICE CUBES)
Calories: 12; Total Fat: <1g; Total Carbs: 3g; Fiber: 1g; Net Carb: 2g; Protein <1g
Macronutrients: Fat: 0%; Protein: 0%; Carbs: 100%

PER SERVING, GINGER-TUMERIC (4 ICE CUBES)
Calories: 4; Total Fat: <1g; Total Carbs: 1g; Fiber: <1g; Net Carbs: 1g; Protein: <1g
Macronutrients: Fat: 0%; Protein: 0%; Carbs: 100%

Garlic- and Chili-Infused Oils

PREP TIME: 5 MINUTES, PLUS 2 HOURS INFUSION TIME | **COOK TIME:** 10 TO 30 MINUTES

I love infusing oils to add a dimension of flavor. The key is to heat the extra-virgin olive oil at a low heat to ensure it doesn't oxidize and take on a rancid flavor. I have found the best temperature for infusing extra-virgin olive oil is 225°F.

GARLIC OIL

**ELIMINATION-FRIENDLY
VEGETARIAN**

CHILI OIL

**NUT- AND SEED-FREE
VEGETARIAN**
MAKES 1 CUP

FOR THE GARLIC OIL

1 cup extra-virgin olive oil
3 garlic cloves, halved

FOR THE CHILI OIL

1 cup extra-virgin olive oil
2 tablespoons red
   pepper flakes

TO MAKE THE GARLIC OIL

1. In a small saucepan, place the olive oil and garlic and heat over low heat.

2. Gently simmer the oil for 30 minutes, making sure it doesn't begin to boil.

3. Pour the mixture into a sealable glass container. Let it sit, covered, at room temperature for an additional 2 hours.

4. Use a slotted spoon to remove the garlic halves and store the oil in the refrigerator for up to 3 days.

TO MAKE THE CHILI OIL

1. In a small saucepan, add the olive oil and heat over medium heat.

2. Once the oil begins to lightly simmer, stir in the red pepper flakes. Immediately turn the heat down to low and heat for 2 to 3 more minutes.

3. Remove from the heat and carefully pour the mixture into a sealable glass container. Let it sit, covered, at room temperature for an additional 2 hours.

4. Store the oil in the refrigerator for up to 3 days.

PER SERVING, GARLIC OIL (2 TABLESPOONS)
Calories: 240; Total Fat: 27g; Total Carbs: 0g; Fiber: 0g; Net Carbs: 0g; Protein: 0g
Macronutrients: Fat: 100%; Protein: 0%; Carbs: 0%

PER SERVING, CHILI OIL (2 TABLESPOONS)
Calories: 242; Total Fat: 27g; Total Carbs: 1g; Fiber: 0g; Net Carbs: 0g; Protein: 0g
Macronutrients: Fat: 99%; Protein: 0%; Carbs: 1%

Homemade Mayonnaise

PREP TIME: 5 MINUTES | **COOK TIME:** 5 MINUTES

Homemade mayonnaise tastes so much better than the store-bought versions you're used to eating! This recipe takes only 10 minutes to make and requires only five ingredients; however, it *does* require an immersion blender.

SUPER-QUICK
ELIMINATION-FRIENDLY
MAKES 1 CUP

1 egg, room temperature
2 teaspoons lemon juice
1 teaspoon Dijon mustard
½ teaspoon pink
   Himalayan salt
1 cup avocado oil

1. Find a tall drinking glass or mason jar wide enough to fit an immersion blender.

2. Gently add the egg to the bottom of the glass, making sure to not break the yolk.

3. Add the lemon juice, Dijon mustard, and salt into the jar. Do *not* stir to combine. Pour the oil into the glass.

4. Place the immersion blender into the glass and submerge it all the way until it hits the bottom.

5. Blend on low power for about 20 seconds without moving the immersion blender.

6. With the immersion blender still on low, slowly start to move the blender up until you reach the top of the oil. Then slowly move the blender back down to the bottom of the glass.

7. Repeat this process, until the mixture thickens and emulsifies.

8. Store in the refrigerator for up to 5 days.

TIP Jazz up this mayo with roasted garlic cloves. To roast garlic, preheat the oven to 400°F. Slice off the top of a whole garlic head and drizzle avocado oil over the exposed cloves. Wrap the garlic head in parchment paper and then wrap with aluminum foil. Roast the garlic for 45 minutes. Remove the garlic head from the oven and cool completely. Squeeze out the individual garlic cloves and add to the glass jar with your lemon juice, mustard, and salt before you pour in the oil.

PER SERVING (1 TABLESPOON)
Calories: 134; Total Fat: 14g; Total Carbs: 0g; Fiber: 0g; Net Carbs: 0g; Protein: <1g
Macronutrients: Fat: 94%; Protein: 6%; Carbs: 0%

Basil Pesto

PREP TIME: 5 MINUTES

Basil pesto is my secret weapon for livening up any keto dish. Add it to scrambled eggs, roasted fish, steamed veggies, or any Italian dish to achieve that next level of flavor.

SUPER-QUICK
VEGETARIAN
MAKES ½ CUP

3 cups fresh basil leaves
2 garlic cloves, halved
¼ cup pine nuts
¼ teaspoon pink
  Himalayan salt
¼ cup extra-virgin olive oil

1. In a food processor, put the basil, garlic, pine nuts, and salt. Process continuously until the ingredients start to break down, about 30 seconds.

2. Slowly pour in the oil and continue to blend until the oil is fully incorporated.

3. Store in a sealed container in the refrigerator for up to 7 days.

TIP You can also freeze the pesto in ice cube trays, transfer the pesto cubes to a zip-top bag, and store them the freezer for up to 6 months.

PER SERVING (2 TABLESPOONS)
Calories: 187; Total Fat: 20g; Total Carbs: 3g; Fiber: 2g; Net Carbs: 1g; Protein: 2g
Macronutrients: Fat: 96%; Protein: 4%; Carbs: 1%

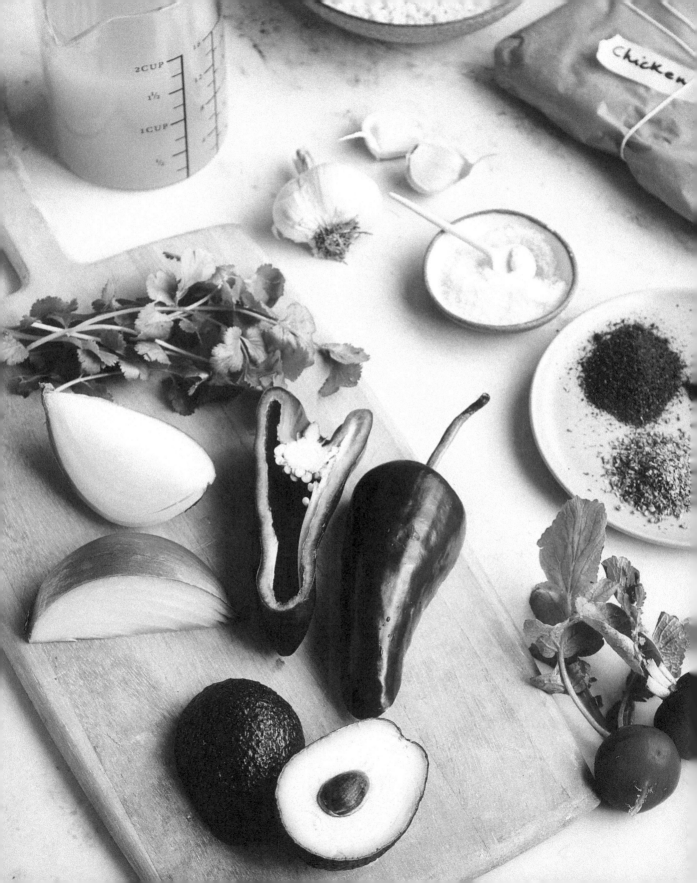

MEASUREMENT CONVERSIONS

VOLUME EQUIVALENTS (LIQUID)

US Standard	US Standard (ounces)	Metric (approximate)
2 tablespoons	1 fl. oz.	30 mL
¼ cup	2 fl. oz.	60 mL
½ cup	4 fl. oz.	120 mL
1 cup	8 fl. oz.	240 mL
1½ cups	12 fl. oz.	355 mL
2 cups or 1 pint	16 fl. oz.	475 mL
4 cups or 1 quart	32 fl. oz.	1 L
1 gallon	128 fl. oz.	4 L

OVEN TEMPERATURES

Fahrenheit (°F)	Celsius (°C) (approximate)
250°F	120°C
300°F	150°C
325°F	165°C
350°F	180°C
375°F	190°C
400°F	200°C
425°F	220°C
450°F	230°C

VOLUME EQUIVALENTS (DRY)

US Standard	Metric (approximate)
⅛ teaspoon	0.5 mL
¼ teaspoon	1 mL
½ teaspoon	2 mL
¾ teaspoon	4 mL
1 teaspoon	5 mL
1 tablespoon	15 mL
¼ cup	59 mL
⅓ cup	79 mL
½ cup	118 mL
⅔ cup	156 mL
¾ cup	177 mL
1 cup	235 mL
2 cups or 1 pint	475 mL
3 cups	700 mL
4 cups or 1 quart	1 L

WEIGHT EQUIVALENTS

US Standard	Metric (approximate)
½ ounce	15 g
1 ounce	30 g
2 ounces	60 g
4 ounces	115 g
8 ounces	225 g
12 ounces	340 g
16 ounces or 1 pound	455 g

REFERENCES

Glick D., S. Barth, and K. F. Macleod. "Autophagy: Cellular and Molecular Mechanisms." *Journal of Pathology* 221, no. 1 (May 2010): 3–12. doi:10.1002/path.2697.

La Merrill, M., C. Emond, M. J. Kim, J-P. Antignac, B. Le Bizec, K. Clément, L. S. Birnbaum, and R. Barouki. "Toxicological Function of Adipose Tissue: Focus on Persistent Organic Pollutants." *Environmental Health Perspectives* 121, 2 (February 2013): 162–9. doi:10.1289/ehp.1205485.

A. Paoli, A. Rubini, J. S. Volek, and K. A. Grimaldi. "Beyond Weight Loss: A Review of the Therapeutic Uses of Very-Low-Carbohydrate (Ketogenic) Diets." *European Journal of Clinical Nutrition* 67 (August 2013): 789–79. doi:10.1038/ejcn.2014.47.

Vojdani, A. "Lectins, Agglutinins, and Their Roles in Autoimmune Reactivities." *Alternative Therapies in Health and Medicine* 21, suppl. 1 (2015): 46–51.

RESOURCES

CleanKetoLifestyle.com: Head over to the official website for more recipes and resources and to connect with me!

Clean Keto Lifestyle: The Complete Guide to Transforming Your Life and Health. My first book is a perfect companion to the *Keto Cleanse.* This book dives into the science behind keto and includes more than 75 keto recipes, five weeks of meal plans, and exercise routines.

The Autoimmune Keto Cookbook: Heal Your Body with Delicious AIP-Compliant Recipes and Meal Plans. This book, written by me and Katie Austin, takes a keto- and Autoimmune Protocol–friendly approach to relieving autoimmune disease symptoms and improving overall well-being. This book has three weeks of meal plans and over 85 delicious recipes.

INDEX

ACKNOWLEDGMENTS

First and foremost, thank you to the amazing team at Rockridge Press for bringing this book to life and being such a joy to work with each day.

To my core support system, including my loving husband, amazing parents and siblings, and the best friends a girl could ask for. You all are the reason I can do what I do and I am beyond grateful you are in my life.

To Katie Austin, my business partner at Clean Keto Lifestyle, for your encouragement in writing this book. You are the most talented chef I know and you have made keto cooking easy, attainable, and *beautiful*!

To the amazing Clean Keto Lifestyle community, who inspires me on a regular basis with your keto success stories, your success energizes me and provided the motivation I needed to spend the long hours writing this book.

ABOUT THE AUTHOR

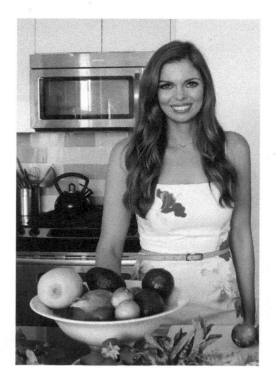

As a global health coach and ketogenic expert, Karissa Long has been living the keto life and helping others live it for almost a decade. She cofounded Clean Keto Lifestyle (CleanKeto-Lifestyle.com), a company focused on helping others achieve their goals through proprietary keto coaching programs, courses, recipes, and meal plans. Karissa found the ketogenic diet during her struggle with ulcerative colitis and has taken everything she learned through her own health journey and made it her mission to help others achieve optimal health.

Karissa is also the bestselling author of *Clean Keto Lifestyle* and coauthor of *The Autoimmune Keto Cookbook*. What makes her method different from other keto programs is that she is all about putting health first and foremost. She focuses on doing the ketogenic diet the right way with a menu free of processed foods and artificial ingredients and full of fresh, clean, nutrient-dense fats, proteins, and vegetables.